# THE
# CORE
# 3 HEALTHY EATING PLAN

## Discover the Simple, Sustainable Way to Lose Weight, Feel Great, and ENJOY FOOD FREEDOM!

**Lisa Moskovitz**, RD, CDN

Adams Media

New York London Toronto Sydney New Delhi

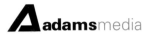

Adams Media
An Imprint of Simon & Schuster, Inc.
100 Technology Center Drive
Stoughton, Massachusetts 02072

First Adams Media trade paperback edition December 2021

ADAMS MEDIA and colophon are trademarks of Simon & Schuster.

For information about special discounts for bulk purchases, please contact Simon & Schuster Special Sales at 1-866-506-1949 or business@simonandschuster.com.

The Simon & Schuster Speakers Bureau can bring authors to your live event. For more information or to book an event contact the Simon & Schuster Speakers Bureau at 1-866-248-3049 or visit our website at www.simonspeakers.com.

Interior design by Colleen Cunningham
Interior photographs by James Stefiuk

Manufactured in the United States of America

1 2021

Library of Congress Cataloging-in-Publication Data
Names: Moskovitz, Lisa, author.
Title: The core 3 healthy eating plan / Lisa Moskovitz, RD, CDN.
Other titles: Core three healthy eating plan
Description: First Adams Media trade paperback edition. | Stoughton, MA: Adams Media, 2021. | Includes index.
Identifiers: LCCN 2021032940 | ISBN 9781507216101 (pb) | ISBN 9781507216118 (ebook)
Subjects: LCSH: Weight loss--Popular works. | Food habits--Psychological aspects. | Exercise--Popular works.
Classification: LCC RM222.2 .M6515 2021 | DDC 613.2/5--dc23
LC record available at https://lccn.loc.gov/2021032940

ISBN 978-1-5072-1610-1
ISBN 978-1-5072-1611-8 (ebook)
1 2021

# Contents

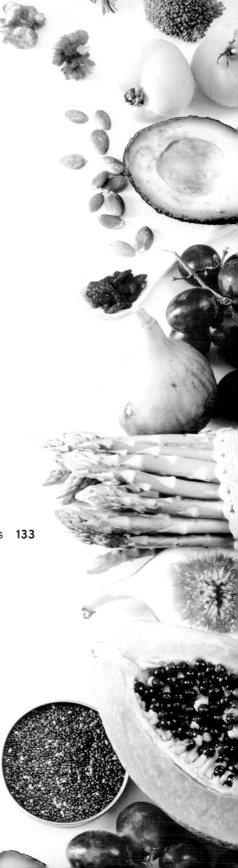

# Preface

**❝I believe a more accurate statistic is that 95 percent of diets fail people.❞**

Ninety-five percent of weight loss diets fail (or so we are told). How is it possible that such an alarming number of diet programs tank, when it seems like everyone around you is losing weight? Your coworker is still thriving after 3 months on the keto diet, and your sister is still proudly tracking Weight Watchers points. I believe a more accurate statistic is that 95 percent of diets fail people. While diets can be effective for short-term weight loss, the majority fizzle out before the 5-month mark. Why? Because these restrictive programs are not personalized, reinforce unhealthy views of food, and are too rigid.

To be successful long-term, you need *structure*, not restrictions. You need to learn how to respect your body's needs and not ignore them with deprivation. That's the foundation of my Core Three Healthy Eating Plan: You'll be able to find your healthiest, happiest weight and/or achieve your healthy eating goals with a science-based plan that doesn't strip you of your autonomy, but rather encourages food freedom.

My experience as a registered dietitian in hospitals and private practices helped me create and refine this plan. Eventually, I built my own private nutrition practice, the NY

Nutrition Group, because I saw the opportunity to serve our clients better. With over fifteen dietitians on staff, we counsel approximately 250-plus clients per week and guide thousands of people toward achieving their optimal health goals with the Core Three formula.

Through my 10-plus years of experience, I have learned valuable insight into what helps and what hurts when it comes to weight management and relationship with food. The Core Three Plan is a product of everything I know and believe will help you lose weight, feel great, and find more food freedom.

I was driven to become a registered dietitian because, like many of my clients, I had my own battles with weight. Like most of yours, mine started in adolescence. I struggled with my relationship with food. I did—and DO—have body image issues to work through. (This work is never done!) I also attempted weight loss at various times in my life because I thought it would bring me happiness. I am not ashamed but rather grateful I had these experiences—I believe they only enhance my qualifications to help others. I not only sympathize with those who come to me for guidance but also empathize with them every step of the way. I understand what it feels like to be where you are right now.

I can proudly say that I am in a much better place than I have ever been before. That's because I went through all the steps of this book myself. I learned, I absorbed, I implemented, and I practiced. Knowledge is power, and I want to empower you to tell the same success story. Anyone can simply follow a diet plan; however, finding your healthiest, happiest weight requires skill. I am living proof of that. And you will be too.

# Introduction

Do you feel discouraged, lost, and confused after repeated failed attempts at weight loss? Do you struggle to figure out what, when, and how to eat? Does your mindset toward food feel obsessive and unhealthy? Are you wondering if it's possible to ever reach your goal weight without starving yourself?

If you're reading this book, your answer is probably yes to all of those questions. *The Core 3 Healthy Eating Plan* is here to help you clear the clutter, debunk dieting myths, and simplify nutrition to make the process intuitive and sustainable. How is this different from any other type of diet book? It is about structure and not restriction. It promotes flexibility, not rigidity. This is not a one-size-fits-all plan that cuts out major food groups, pushes products, or strips you of your autonomy. The Core Three employs the number *three* throughout the plan for several reasons. Not only does it make it easier to remember and implement, but thinking in threes is the simple, scientific solution to find a balanced, healthy lifestyle. The plan also provides a three-step approach to finding your healthiest, happiest weight including a meal plan built around the Core Three macronutrients: high-fiber carbohydrates, lean proteins, and anti-inflammatory fats. Three also represents a past, present, and future. Your past may be riddled with failed

> **❝** Thinking in threes is the simple, scientific solution to find a balanced, healthy lifestyle. **❞**

diet attempts and weight struggles, but you are presently finding a real solution for a much more fulfilling, successful future. The premise of the Meals and Hydration portion of the Core Three is simple: Incorporate the three major macronutrients—the trifecta—in the portions necessary to fuel (without overfueling) your body and keep blood sugar levels stable. While we don't count calories, we do pay attention to eating a balance of nutritious food groups. The key elements of the plan are as follows:

| **Core Three Meals and Hydration** | <ul><li>**Eat every *three* hours** (or four) throughout the day.</li><li>**Include at least *three* servings of each of the *three* core macronutrients per day:**<ul><li>High-fiber carbohydrate</li><li>Lean protein</li><li>Anti-inflammatory fat</li></ul></li><li>**Add at least *three* servings of non-starchy vegetables per day.**</li><li>**Drink up to *three* liters of water per day.**</li></ul> |
| --- | --- |
| **Core Three Exercise** | <ul><li>**Exercise moderately *three* hours per week.**</li></ul> |
| **Core Three Tracking Method** | <ul><li>**Journal your food for a minimum of *three* days per week**, or just the first *three* months of starting your journey.</li><li>**Weigh yourself only *three* times each month** (or four), preferably using body composition analysis.</li><li>**Track your progress for *three* weeks** before making any adjustments.</li></ul> |

The Core Three Healthy Eating Plan respects the need for personalization and flexibility, along with a healthy relationship with food and your body. It can be adapted not just for weight loss but also for blood sugar control, hormonal imbalance, improved cholesterol, healthier gut, and long-term weight maintenance once you find your healthiest, happiest weight. *The Core 3 Healthy Eating Plan* will help you:

- Heal your relationship with your body.
- Discover your eating archetype and remedies to improve your relationship with food.
- Learn the nutrition fundamentals so you can become a healthier, more confident eater.
- Develop a plan—using the *three* core macronutrients—to find your happiest, healthiest weight.
- Understand why *three* hours of exercise per week is ideal for health and weight management.
- Acquire skills, like food journaling at least *three* times per week, to guarantee success.
- Adapt the plan for special conditions like polycystic ovary syndrome (PCOS), hypothyroidism, diabetes, eating disorders, and postmenopausal and postpartum body changes that can cause barriers to healthy body image and healthy eating.
- Prepare meals with more than fifty easy-to-follow healthy recipes and a variety of meal plans.
- Access a private Facebook group with additional recipes, tips, and support.

This book is divided into *three* parts:

**1** **The first part** is to start healing your relationship with food and your body. Weight loss does not automatically improve body image, which is why it's important to learn strategies to feel more satisfied with, and proud of, the skin you're in.

**2** **The second part** is to understand the Core Three way of eating. This is where we will explore the Core Three macronutrients, the role they play, and how they fuel your body for healthy weight loss. In this part, you will find helpful tables that detail foods and serving sizes for each of the macronutrients.

**3**    **The third part** is to learn how to personalize, adapt, and maintain the Core Three Plan to fit your specific needs and preferences. Along with this personalization, I will teach you the necessary skills for long-term success. You will also find more than fifty recipes and several structured plans to help guide your meal choices.

It may be tempting to race right to the meal plan portion of the book if you're eager to lose weight. However, without reading through all three parts first, you will not understand the relevance and importance of how this plan is laid out.

It's time to break free of quick-fix weight loss diets that only cause stress to your body. Wouldn't it feel great to eat *for* your body instead of fighting *against* it? With the Core Three's all-inclusive, whole food–based approach, you will finally find food freedom. You can trust that you are receiving the value of nutrition counseling from a registered dietitian who has seen what it takes for long-term success. *The Core 3 Healthy Eating Plan* is the last "diet" book you'll ever have to read to discover the simple, sustainable way to lose weight, feel great, and enjoy food freedom!

# 1

# BEFORE YOU START THE PLAN

CHAPTER 1

# How Is Your Relationship with Your Body?

The Core Three encourages more freedom with your food choices. But to feel free with your eating, you must first feel free in your body. To feel free in your body, it is important to develop a healthier relationship with your body. The fundamentals of any healthy relationship include respect, trust, and appreciation, but do you have that with your body? How often do you look in the mirror and respect what you see? How often do you trust your body to guide your food choices? How much time do you spend appreciating and nourishing your body instead of trying to change it?

The truth is, losing weight will not automatically improve your body image. That's part of the reason the Core Three Healthy Eating Plan is not *just* about weight loss. A healthier relationship with your body materializes when you stop believing weight loss is the solution to all your body image battles.

In this chapter, we'll explore how to work through body image issues before beginning the Core Three Plan. I will dive into the origins of body image issues so that you can identify the signs. I'll provide you with concrete tips to improve your relationship with your body, including certain self-care habits and how to find a new happy weight. I'll help you understand why you shouldn't rely on the body mass index (BMI) and why measuring body composition is a more accurate way to track your progress. Feeling good in your skin is a journey, and this chapter is the first step.

## The Body Image Struggle Is Real

What is body image? Simply put, it's how you view *and feel in* your body. A healthy body image means that you feel comfortable and confident in the skin you are in. You might not love it all the time, but you appreciate it. A negative body image, or unhealthy relationship with your body, can lead to a multitude of problems, including mental health issues, poor quality of life, and a dysfunctional relationship with food. Body image struggles can originate from early life experiences and be exacerbated by genetics, environmental stimuli, and mental or physical ailments.

### Did a Childhood Experience Cause Your Body Image Issues?

Most people develop a negative body image at a young age. According to the National Eating Disorders Association (NEDA), weight concerns begin by age six! Body image issues often start after someone is teased about their appearance by other kids, compares themselves to models and celebrities, or goes to a routine checkup with a pediatrician who prescribes weight loss for a healthier BMI-for-age percentile.

Parents and family members are by far the most influential sources for your self-image. Even if well intentioned, parents who put their child on a diet or withhold food to encourage weight loss are sending a message to their child that their appearance is unacceptable. I have adult clients who complain that their parents *still* make comments about their appearance, food choices, or weight changes. Whether it's a compliment or a criticism, the constant emphasis on weight and body can be irrevocable.

If someone tells you that you need to lose weight for years on end, whether or not that's true, you're going to believe it. Over time, this "you're not good enough" feedback will chip away at your self-esteem, health, and happiness. On the flip side, if you received constant praise for your appearance, and then the compliments eventually stopped as you got older, it could also have significant repercussions. This is something that happened to me. I played soccer for years—peers would often remark about my size and muscle tone. Eventually when I stopped playing sports, I started noticing changes in my body. Due to the drastic decline in activity, my clothes started getting tighter, my tummy felt softer, and my self-confidence diminished. It felt like I'd lost my identity as the small athletic girl and was suddenly more curvaceous. Of course, being curvy is not bad, but when a physical change happens suddenly, it can feel like a real identity crisis. Fears of judgment, scrutiny of your physical appearance, and pity can be debilitating.

In either scenario, the attachment to a body size and how that affects self-confidence is the underpinning issue. Before you attempt to improve how you look on the outside, you need to work on how you feel on the inside. Sure, it may be easier to feel good about how you look after you lose weight, but true beauty is always an inside job.

## The Diet Culture That Bombards Us

Diet culture can be defined as how society glorifies being thin and equates thinness with a measure of success and value. Living in this environment affects the way we feel about our bodies. Social media, influencers, the fashion industry, advertisers, celebrities, and even certain medical professionals can perpetuate the "thin ideal." This overarching message significantly influences the way you feel about yourself and your body satisfaction. Talking negatively about your body is normalized, even *expected* in certain situations. Diets and weight loss are common topics of conversation at social gatherings. Diet culture can be overt or sneaky—but it is certainly ubiquitous. It affects people of all ages, races, incomes, religions, genders, and ethnicities. Understanding and recognizing it is the first step to desensitizing yourself to its toxicity.

Next time you're with family and your aunt confesses, "I'm so bad for eating that chocolate cake," recognize that this is diet culture. When your friend walks into the room and everyone immediately compliments her recent weight loss, that's diet culture. And when you believe that your weight or size is the reason you're single or didn't get that dream job, that's diet culture leading you to doubt your self-worth.

### Body Image and Medical Issues

If you have ever experienced any medical issues that add stress to, and considerably complicate, your day-to-day life, then accepting and appreciating your body can prove more difficult. These can present as chronic bloating and digestion issues that make it hard to eat out, socialize, and feel confident in your clothes or as much more life-threatening, debilitating chronic conditions such as diabetes or cancers. What it boils down to is that while medical issues can absolutely make it much harder to feel your best and appreciate your body, focusing on self-care is even more important for your health and happiness. Although medical issues can certainly impede your ability to practice self-care, prepare and cook meals, or exercise, understanding that you are still worth the investment is a part of total body acceptance.

Most body image discussion centers on weight stigmas, but it is not uncommon to feel body dissatisfaction for a multitude of reasons that have nothing to do with weight whatsoever. For example, people who realize that their gender does not align with the one they were assigned at birth may struggle to feel as though their image fits in with society's narrow view of what's "acceptable." Appreciating the body blueprint you were born with can prove challenging for other populations too.

## When Weight Is a Health Issue

Of course, weight loss is not just about feeling better in jeans or a bathing suit. Losing weight can affect more than aesthetics and appearance. Countless studies attest to the long-term health implications of excess weight or body fat. According to the Centers for Disease Control and Prevention (CDC), if you're considered "obese" on the BMI chart, losing just 5–10 percent of your total body weight can improve blood pressure, blood cholesterol, and blood sugar levels. Further, the National Weight Control Registry noted that "study participants who achieved a healthier weight for their height" reported better energy levels, physical mobility, general mood, and self-confidence. In the United States, obesity is associated with the leading causes of preventable death—it is linked to heart disease, diabetes, and cancer. An estimated 300,000 deaths per year are due to the obesity epidemic. *That said, weight loss can certainly increase chances of a healthier, longer life—as long as it's achieved using a healthy approach.*

Weight-related health issues are not exclusive to those who are overweight. The pressure to control weight and to avoid some of the previously listed obesity-related health complications can lead to other problems as well. Unhealthy, restrictive diets coupled with immense weight gain fears can spark eating disorders. Eating disorders have the second highest mortality rate of all mental health disorders, surpassed only by substance use disorders, as revealed by a 2014 meta-review in the peer-reviewed journal *World Psychiatry*. Prioritizing weight loss over health leads to a myriad of problems that can be just as detrimental as the problems associated with obesity, if not more so.

## Signs of an Unhealthy Body Image

How do you find a balance between accepting your body and wanting to improve it? Is it possible to attempt weight loss without developing an unhealthy attitude about your weight? Most anti-diet activists believe that dieting and any intentional weight loss is pointless, even a danger. They preach that the only way to improve body image is to rid our society of all diet talk entirely. First, this is not realistic. Whether it's a body image issue or not, we all want to feel great and confident in our clothes (or without our clothes). And without a doubt, it is easier to be body positive when you're in a smaller body. Second, we know that intentional weight loss can have its benefits. No one should feel bad about wanting to feel their best. So where is the happy medium? It's in making sure your intentions remain positive and that you are not sacrificing your mental health for your physical appearance.

### Get a Helping Hand

While you can jump-start your progress with the steps in this book, if your body struggles are significantly impacting your life, it may be best to hire a professional. A therapist and/or dietitian can guide you through the healing process. Either way, know that you are doing a lot and you are enough.

Here are some signs of an unhealthy relationship with your body and tips on finding more balance:

**You weigh yourself on a scale frequently and attach your weight to your self-worth.** Weighing in on a scale is the most common way to track progress. However, weighing yourself too frequently can *cause* body image issues, especially when you rely on the number you see for validation—if you notice your weight has gone up, you immediately feel like a failure; if your weight goes down, you instantly feel proud or "acceptable."

Don't give the scale that much power. First, know that the scale lies and your body is predominantly water, so weight fluctuations are often related to just that. Second, if the scale does affect your mindset, try alternative methods of tracking (which will be discussed later in this chapter and more in Chapter 11).

**You avoid certain social situations (like pool parties) for fear of judgment.** No matter where you go or who you are with, remember that everyone is dealing with their own insecurities. You are not alone. If you are worried about people judging you, chances are they are worried about your judgement too. The reality is that no one is judging your body more than you are. Get outside of your head, but first, ask yourself, "Do I really care what a person thinks of me if they are that quick to judge me based on the size of my clothes and the shape of my legs?" Quite frankly, anyone who makes you feel bad about the way you look is not worth your time (and is probably projecting).

**You do not enjoy exercising or moving your body.** When you view exercise as a requirement to lose weight or use it to compensate for overeating, it is not going to feel like an enjoyable activity. You are placing too much pressure on yourself and associating exercise with punishment. In Chapter 8, I will explain how to use exercise as a reward, not a punishment. Moving mindfully and focusing on improving physical strength through exercise versus burning fat can instantly improve the way you view your body. You will find a new appreciation for moving your body and for how you look and feel.

**You often scrutinize your appearance in the mirror, focusing only on your perceived flaws.** Just because you *think* your body looks a certain way, that doesn't mean it's true. Practice positive affirmations to overrule any negative thinking patterns. Write down how often you look in the mirror and criticize your appearance in 1 week. Add it up and think about ALL the other things you could be doing with that time. Wouldn't you rather finish refurbishing that dresser, knit that blanket for your nephew, or write that blog post than ruminate over your arms? In fact, make a list of activities that would bring more meaning and joy to your life and post it over your mirror as a reprioritization reminder. Here's one example: "Stop looking at your thighs and start looking for a more fulfilling job!"

**You are significantly more motivated to eat "healthy" and exercise for weight loss rather than to improve your health.** Sure, eating a balanced, nutrient-dense diet; engaging in moderate exercise; and prioritizing sleep can result in healthy weight loss. However, the real incentive is that investing in these self-care behaviors supports your immune system, balances your hormones, strengthens your heart, improves your mood, and boosts gut health. Shift your focus from how food changes the outside of your body to how food helps the inside of your body. When you devote time and attention to improving your health on a deeper level, it can instantly boost your self-confidence and body image satisfaction—especially when you realize a healthy body image starts from within.

**It takes you a long time to pick out an outfit in the morning or before going out.** Clothes come in a variety of shapes, colors, and sizes. They are designed to fit your body, not the other way around. You don't have to wear clothes just because they're trendy. Dress for your body, and only dress up for yourself. It's great to have an appreciation for fashion, but if that interferes with your self-worth and body acceptance, then it's just not worth it. Confidence comes from within, and your clothes should reflect that. When they do, it's easy to pick out an outfit you feel great in!

**You frequently compare your body to others' bodies.** Remember that "the grass is always greener." The person you might *think* has it better than you may actually be struggling even more than you are. To reframe your thinking, remember everything you have to be thankful for in your life. (You can even start a gratitude journal, which is recommended in Chapter 11.) It may also help to evaluate who you follow on social media. Platforms like Instagram and TikTok are notorious for igniting a comparison spiral. Take social media breaks and consider following only accounts that make you feel better about yourself, like body-positive advocates and influencers.

**You feel uncomfortable in your body most of the time.** The key word here is "feel." Not feeling good about the way you look is clearly a symptom that your body image is in a negative place. But feeling this way might be related to a deeper emotion. You might actually feel anxious, upset, or lonely, but you're expressing that through a physical judgment. There are many understandable reasons to be in a negative headspace: a fight with your partner, negative feedback from a supervisor, or a triggering post on social media. Don't brush off these uncomfortable emotions or triggers; deal with them instead, maybe by reaching out to supportive friends or family, going for a walk, journaling, enjoying a hot bath, or just taking a minute to reflect. If you're sad, it's okay to cry. If you're angry, it's okay to let that out too. Otherwise, you could be translating other disappointments into a negative body image. Remember, body image is not just about what we see in the mirror. It is also how we *feel* about what we see.

**You impulsively reject compliments about your physical appearance.** If you feel uncomfortable accepting compliments, you can practice on yourself so it feels more natural. The more you give yourself positive feedback and praise, the more you will believe in your self-worth. Practicing self-acceptance also opens you up to accepting compliments from others. Know that you are worth more than your weight and deserve to be happy despite what the scale says. There is no perfect body shape, and your weight is the *least* interesting thing about you. Recognize all of your enviable internal and external qualities.

If even one or two of these behaviors resonate, then your body image has likely interfered with your well-being.

### Respect Isn't Reserved for Smaller Bodies

"But Lisa, it's so much easier to respect, love, and appreciate your body when it's smaller." I frequently hear this from clients, and you might agree, but I promise that losing weight will not help you suddenly develop a fondness for your legs, arms, or abs. That has to come from *within*. In fact, I am a firm believer that you must feel love on the inside before you can see it on the outside. Healing your relationship with your body will make your wellness process and Core Three journey much easier and more productive.

It is crucial to recognize that you and your body are a team. To feel your best, you must work with it—not against it—through self-compassion and self-care. You have plenty of positive qualities and strengths, but a pathological worry about your weight, body, and appearance will blunt your potential. Be gentle and patient with yourself as you change your habits and behaviors—body image healing is a journey, and change will take time.

## A Healthy Body Image Cannot Be Reduced to One Number

Part of loving your body is reevaluating your goal or ideal weight. What if your dream weight is actually a dangerous weight? Instead, aim for a happy weight. Your happy weight is the RANGE of numbers you feel your best at. A happy weight is the point between appreciating your body and wanting to make changes so you can feel your best. It may not be your ideal BMI, or the ideal weight that shows up when you Google "what is the healthiest weight for my height." It is subjective and cannot be reduced to a single predetermined number. Here's another tip: *Your happiest weight isn't the least you've ever weighed.* In Chapter 11, I will explain how to find your happiest, healthiest weight. For now, just know that your relationship with the numbers on the scale will likely be different than it's been in the past and

that you will want to try to separate your body image from a certain number on the scale.

### The Problem with the BMI

Even if you look beyond your weight, society has other "numbers" it wants you to focus on…and those are problematic too. The BMI is simply a measurement of your weight in kilograms divided by your height in meters squared. The more you weigh, the higher your BMI will be. A "healthy" BMI is considered 18.5–24.9, while 25–29.9 is "overweight" and 30 or greater is "obese."

The truth is, this 200-year-old artifact was created by a mathematician, not a medical expert. It originated as a formula for government officials to use when allocating resources. Not only was it designed centuries ago, but this marginalizing tool also doesn't account for body composition, waist size, sex, or body type. For that reason, I will ask you to consider a better method to track progress and stay healthy: body composition.

### Body Composition: A More Reliable Tracking System

While using any set of weight-related numbers to determine success can harm body image, it is also difficult to determine how you're responding to a plan without some type of measurement. For that reason, body composition is a more reliable way to measure progress than the BMI chart, the total number on the scale, or even the size of your clothes. Your body composition refers to how much of your total weight is body fat versus muscle. It will tell you your body fat percentage and even how many pounds of muscle and water you have. Seeing total pounds increase on the scale is not nearly as discouraging when you notice it's mostly in the form of water or, even better, muscle! You can find user-friendly body composition devices online to purchase for your home. And many fitness facilities and dietitians have larger, more advanced measuring devices available to use as needed.

### The Set Point Theory of Weight

The Set Point Theory is based on the understanding that most individuals have a certain predetermined weight that is their genetic blueprint. No matter how hard you try, you may find yourself back to the same range of pounds on the scale or clothing size. This doesn't mean you are sentenced to an unhappy weight. Your DNA might be the genetic blueprint, but you're still the builder who holds the artistic license. It just helps to understand that if you have been struggling for the majority of your life to maintain a smaller size, it's might not be your fault. You either have not found the right plan yet or have pushed your body too far. That's okay! You still have options to feel your healthiest.

One of the most important takeaways from this chapter is that losing weight will not automatically improve your body image. You must team up with your body to find that balance between improving and respecting your body at the same time. This is the best approach to finding your healthiest, happiest weight. A healthier relationship with your body lays the foundation for a healthy relationship with food, which we will discuss in the next chapter.

# CHAPTER 2

# How Is Your Relationship with Food?

A positive relationship with food is the hallmark of the Core Three Healthy Eating Plan. A healthy food connection requires respect, appreciation, and trust, the tenets of any good relationship. Do you respect, appreciate, and trust food?

In this chapter, we'll evaluate your relationship with food and determine if it requires rehabilitation. We will touch upon disordered eating and the different ways it develops. I will introduce "The Four Distorted Eater Archetypes," what defines them, and how to work through them to achieve a healthier relationship with food. These strategies include mindful eating, recognizing real hunger versus emotional hunger, identifying "food triggers," and challenging "food rules." The tools you acquire in this chapter will heal your relationship with food and help set you up for Core Three success.

## Assessing Your Relationship with Food

We all need food to live, but you might not spend much time thinking about your relationship with this vital substance. Take a few moments now to reflect on your beliefs around eating and how food fits into your life.

### Do You Have a Healthy Relationship with Food?

A healthy relationship with food means feeling free with your food choices. This can look different for each person, but these are the main hallmarks:

- You see food as a source of nourishment and fuel.
- You allow yourself a variety of foods. There are no "good" and "safe" nor "bad" and "feared" foods.
- Hunger is a natural feeling you recognize and respect.
- You enjoy eating, but it is not your only source of pleasure.
- You don't let stress, or other emotions, dictate food choices—whether that means overeating or undereating.
- You don't try to control your eating or deny yourself food.
- If you overeat, you don't feel the need to compensate with exercise or food restriction.
- You eat as mindfully as possible.

### Do You Have an Unhealthy Relationship with Food?

On the opposite end of the spectrum, an unhealthy relationship with food can often stem from body dissatisfaction, which leads to chronic dieting or other drastic eating habits to "change" your body shape or size. Your relationship with food is likely tied to how it makes you feel:

- If food makes you feel anxious, eating food will make you feel anxious.
- If you think certain foods are "bad," then you will feel "bad" eating those foods.
- If you are constantly worried about overeating, you may feel like you eat too much.

When untreated, a poor relationship with food can segue into an eating disorder, which warrants multidisciplinary medical attention. According to NEDA, "eating disorders are serious but treatable mental and physical illnesses that can affect people of all genders, ages, races, religions, ethnicities, sexual orientations, body shapes, and weights." They are diagnosed by medical professionals. Before it gets to that point, there are often signs of less complicated distorted eating. Identifying certain behaviors or characteristics is the first step to improve your relationship with food and, most importantly, help prevent life-altering eating disorders.

## The Four Distorted Eater Archetypes

Your relationship with food is personal and usually develops key characteristics. Some people know their food issues already; others need to raise their awareness of what and how they eat in order to identify the problems.

I believe that most people who struggle with their food relationship will relate to at least one of these four archetypes:

1. The Erratic Eater
2. The Dependent Eater
3. The Judgmental Eater
4. The Obsessive Eater

While there are some differences between these four archetypes, there are also several commonalities: All archetypes struggle to identify and properly respond to hunger and fullness cues. Most people in each of the archetypes are aware that issues with food exist, but they do not yet have the tools to work through them. Most, if not all, find it difficult to find and maintain a healthy, happy weight. Let's take a deeper look at the four archetypes and learn how to work through specific pitfalls related to each.

### The Erratic Eater

Erratic Eaters rarely have a daily eating routine, which can contribute to poor habits and poor nutritional intake.

### CHARACTERISTIC BEHAVIORS

- Distracted, mindless eating
- Fast-paced eating, often finishing meals before their companions
- Consuming large quantities of food later in the day after quasi-fasting
- Nighttime or after-dinner snacking

### THE PITFALLS OF THE ERRATIC EATER

- Nutritionally imbalanced food choices, as their meals tend to be quick and convenient
- High risk of undereating and/or overeating
- Stress or anxious feelings leading to appetite suppression and then subsequent overeating
- Digestion issues like bloating or acid reflux
- Fluctuating blood sugars due to inconsistent eating times

Remedies for Erratic Eaters include planning ahead and eating more mindfully.

### SOLUTION
### PLAN AHEAD

It's okay if you're not the three-meals-per-day type, but take time to plan. Stock up on nutrient-dense foods so that they are more accessible. Plan meals with a variety of food groups. A little thinking ahead will go a long way in improving your relationship with food.

## MAKE MEALS MORE MINDFUL

Mindful eating is not a weight loss technique, but mindless eating can certainly lead to overeating and unnecessary weight gain. Mindful eating is conscious eating and involves total awareness. Paying attention to the food in front of you can increase satisfaction and food appreciation. Make sure to focus on your food—not the social media on your phone. Engage your senses involving the taste and texture of what you're eating. Take the time to actually sit down and eat instead of shoveling food into your mouth while hovering over the kitchen counter. Again, mindful eating is not about eating less, but you will be more satisfied and less likely to eat past what your body requires for fuel.

Mindful eating is the most natural way to portion out your meals. You don't need a measuring cup, food scale, phone app, or fancy tracking device to determine what your body needs. If you slow down and pay attention, your body will tell you. While eating on the Core Three Plan, it's important to practice mindful eating. The more you practice, the more natural it will feel. Chew slowly, or at least twenty times before swallowing; put your fork down in between bites; and even put on some relaxing music to set the mood. Here is a mindful eating exercise to try at home:

1. Select a finger food like pretzels, grapes, or cheese cubes.
2. Find a calm, quiet environment and have a seat.
3. Pick up the food and observe. Take notice of its shape, color, and surfaces.
4. Bring the food closer to your nose. How does it smell?
5. Place the food in your mouth. How does it feel and taste?
6. Start chewing and pause to notice taste and texture.
7. Chew thoroughly before swallowing.

When you finish eating, reflect:

- Was it enjoyable?
- How was this experience different from how you normally eat?
- Did anything surprise you?
- What did you notice in terms of sight, touch, sound, smell, and taste?
- What thoughts or memories popped up?
- What do you want to take from this experience for your future eating habits?

## The Dependent Eater

Dependent Eaters may use food as a coping mechanism for uncomfortable emotions but also to celebrate, reward, and incentivize actions. While eating is meant to be pleasurable, if food is the only source of pleasure, it is problematic.

### CHARACTERISTIC BEHAVIORS

- Compulsively consuming food based on social and environmental cues, such

as needing popcorn at the movies or a pastry when walking by a bakery
- Eating more food if it's in front of them, especially if others are doing so
- Usually planning activities that involve some type of food or eating
- Overpacking snacks whenever going anywhere to prevent feeling hungry
- Potentially binge-eating

### THE PITFALLS OF THE DEPENDENT EATER
- Neglected and suppressed emotions or, alternatively, persistent guilt or depression
- A higher intake of sugary, salty, or pro-inflammatory fat-rich foods
- Difficultly maintaining weight and blood sugar levels

You can remedy these issues by recognizing when you are overeating, understanding the difference between physical and emotional hunger, and identifying your eating triggers.

### SOLUTION

### OVERCOME OVEREATING

Overeating means eating more than your body requires to function or more than it is burning. If you feel uncomfortably full after meals, bloated, sluggish, or just unwell, it is possible you are overeating.

Overcoming overeating first requires eating balanced meals at regular intervals to regulate blood sugars and appetite.

The Core Three Healthy Eating Plan will provide you personalized guidelines to use while fine-tuning your hunger and fullness cues. The longer you wait to eat, the harder it becomes to respond to your hunger sensibly and mindfully and to stop when you're comfortably satisfied rather than uncomfortably full. Try the mindful eating exercise in the "Solution: Make Meals More Mindful" section earlier in this chapter to help slow your eating pace.

You may want to figure out why you have these overeating episodes. Many external factors could be causing you to overeat, including boredom, fatigue, hormones, stress, and just the presence of food. Find non-food-related means to process these emotions. Here are some alternatives to bypass nonphysiological hunger:

- Distract yourself. Go for a walk, stretch, or take a hot bath. A few minutes of a relaxing activity can boost feel-good neurotransmitters that mitigate the urge to eat.
- Call a friend or family member. Talking to supportive and comforting people you love can fill the emotional void driving you to eat.
- Journal your emotions. It is free and therapeutic, and it off-loads feelings you may be struggling to process. Emotional eating occurs for the same reason.
- Find a new hobby. Enjoyable activities that are also challenging offer a sense of accomplishment. This can satisfy

you on a deeper level, replacing the need to snack or eat sweets.

- Seek professional help. A professional such as a therapist or dietitian can provide the individual attention you need to manage whatever life throws your way.

**DIFFERENTIATE BETWEEN PHYSIOLOGICAL AND EMOTIONAL HUNGER**

Hunger is innate, driving us to satisfy a need for fuel (physiological) and nourishment but also a need for comfort (emotional). It is common to eat when you're really just hungry for human connection. Here is what true physiological hunger can look like:

- Low energy levels, or fatigue, due to decreased blood sugar
- Stomach pains due to churning stomach acids
- Difficulty concentrating due to lack of nutrients—your brain requires food to function
- Irritability or mood swings, which are related to dips in blood sugar
- Dizziness or light-headedness due decreasing blood pressure

When you feel an urge to eat, ask:

- When was the last time I ate? Was it more than 3 hours ago?
- Am I tired? Would I rather have a nap?
- Am I tense, anxious, or bored? Can I do something else instead?

- How hungry am I? On a scale of 1–10 (10 being ravenous), if you're at a 4 or lower, find a distraction. If you're above that, eat. Resisting may backfire.

**IDENTIFY YOUR EATING TRIGGERS**

Eating triggers are circumstances or environments that cause you to seek food. These experiences can bring up uncomfortable emotions or memories. They can often be linked to past traumas that cause distress. Triggers can be unavoidable, so it's critical to reflect on why you respond in certain ways and how to better manage them.

Dr. Marsha Linehan is an American psychologist and the creator of dialectical behavior therapy (DBT), a type of psychotherapy that treats various mental health disorders through behavioral science, acceptance, and mindfulness. Dr. Linehan created the STOP skill, which was designed to help overcome distress and prevent further damage. I have adapted her original premise to address food triggers:

- **S**top and avoid reacting with emotions that drive other harmful, impulsive behaviors. Name the emotion in that triggering moment.
- **T**ake a step back. Give yourself time and distance to process your emotions in a calm environment. Do an activity that is soothing, like talking to someone, going for a walk, or washing dishes.

- **O**bserve your surroundings. It will help you refocus and remain present.
- **P**roceed mindfully and gather more information. Ask yourself, "What outcome do I want from this situation?" Your brain needs time to handle the triggering event without turning to food.

### The Judgmental Eater

This type of eater is chronically labeling food as "good" or "bad." Judgmental Eaters often criticize their own food choices and may even project these criticisms onto others. Years of chronic dieting contribute to such polarizing food views and repeated self-judgement.

#### CHARACTERISTIC BEHAVIORS

- Quickly believing what they read or hear regarding nutrition and health in the news
- Thriving on rules, structure, and an authoritarian approach toward eating—unable to see nuance
- Taking an all-or-nothing approach to dieting

#### THE PITFALLS OF THE JUDGMENTAL EATER

- Feeling like a failure because of high and/or unrealistic expectations
- Metabolic decline, muscle loss, and nutritional deficiencies as a result of abuse from yo-yo dieting and weight loss cycling

- Little body trust and overuse of scale to track weight
- Overeating, as demonizing foods puts them on a pedestal
- Trigger eating

Remedy these issues by overcoming food rules and rigid attitudes about food.

**SOLUTION**

#### EXAMINE AND CHALLENGE FOOD RULES

Food rules are eating stipulations enforced by diet plans or authority figures. They shape attitudes and beliefs surrounding eating. Examples include:

**Myth: Stop eating after 6:00 p.m.**
**Truth:** Eating after 6:00 p.m. doesn't automatically equate to weight gain, especially if you are active at night and have a later bedtime. Generally, a 2- or 3-hour window between your last meal and slumber is sufficient for proper digestion.

**Myth: Avoid all processed, packaged foods.**
**Truth:** While certain ultraprocessed foods may not be as nutritious as minimally processed foods, processing can be quite beneficial in certain situations. It makes a variety of foods available and safe for consumption. Whole-grain cereals, baby carrots, canned tuna and beans, and frozen veggies are all technically packaged or processed foods that are incredibly nutritious and convenient.

**Myth: Eat fewer than 1,200 calories for weight loss.**
**Truth:** Exercise, activity level, body composition, and metabolic rate all determine your caloric needs. With the exception of those under age three or over age ninety-three, most people need well over 1,200 calories for proper nutrient absorption and energy and to keep up with physical demands. Undereating can also slow down your metabolism over time.

**Myth: Gluten and dairy are bad for you.**
**Truth:** Sure, if your diet is mostly pizza, ice cream, and bagels with cream cheese, you may feel better after cutting out these foods. However, not everyone is sensitive to gluten and dairy specifically. If you suspect an allergy or intolerance, consult with a medical professional before omitting major food groups.

**Myth: All carbs cause weight gain.**
**Truth:** Chapter 4 will cover all the reasons why this is not true. While carbs can increase body fat over time, it all depends on how many and which type of carbs you're eating.

Of course, everyone is different, and some of you may find following food rules to be beneficial. The issue is that most rules around food can damage your relationship with food. Rules often exacerbate Judgmental Eating and make it difficult to enjoy meals. If you're constantly worried about not eating certain foods, chances are that all you will think about is the food you're supposed to avoid. You are no longer present and are disconnected from hunger and fullness cues. Fight against food rules and replace them with internal eating awareness. For example, if you've always believed that you can't have bread with dinner, ask yourself, "Do I really feel any different when I have a little bread with dinner?" Maybe you feel more satisfied and snack less at night when it's included in the meal. Question what's real and what's simply a distorted food belief. Beliefs are often just reoccurring thoughts that we picked up somewhere or from someone. Come up with a new list that is based on understanding your body. Everyone is different, and the only one who can tell you the best way to eat for you is YOU.

**SOLUTION**

**RESIST RIGID ATTITUDES ABOUT FOOD**
Food choices are influenced by many factors, both external and internal, including environment, culture, convenience, time, diet plans, electronics, social media, people, emotions, knowledge, energy, hormones, and activity level. However, one of the biggest motivators in eating is how it makes you look and feel. If your goal is to lose weight, you are probably making food choices based on that goal—even if those run counter to what your body is asking for. You might say to yourself, "I should eat this" or "I should not eat that." However,

*should*-ing yourself can wreak havoc on your relationship with food. Challenge the "should" with "would" and "could." If you immediately think, "I *should* order the side of broccoli instead of French fries," follow that with "I *would* be more satisfied with the French fries, so I *could* have a little bit of both." Compromising will satisfy both your wants and needs.

Rigidity is not a sign of willpower. It leads to rebellion and an all-or-nothing attitude toward eating that can eventually implode your weight loss efforts. You're either all-in "on a diet" or doing nothing "off a diet." You are stuck in a cycle of scolding yourself and then rebelling against this ineffective attempt at control. You become increasingly disconnected from physiological hunger cues, which can trigger overeating. Compromising with food choices, adapting to each situation, and working through anxious or guilty feelings are essential ingredients to a more functional relationship with food.

## SOLUTION

### STOP FORBIDDING FOODS

A healthy relationship with food balances nutrient-dense with discretionary foods. Discretionary foods are not necessarily nutritious, but they add enjoyment and variety. Chocolate is not a core food group, but it can still be a part of a healthy diet. However, if discretionary foods replace nutrient-dense foods, that's a different story. The Core Three focuses on what to *add* to your diet, not what to take out. Adding lean proteins, high-fiber carbohydrates, and anti-inflammatory fats will naturally crowd out other foods without completely excluding them.

When you say something is off-limits, it instantly becomes more appealing—you want what you can't have. You also send a message to yourself that *you have no self-control and can't be trusted around particular foods.* This is why food-forbidding often results in the exact opposite of the desired effect—you end up with stronger, harder-to-suppress cravings. Instead, challenge yourself to keep these foods around, enjoy them, and accept that you need to be flexible with your eating habits. Store them out of sight so that they are not as accessible as fresh fruit, veggies, nuts, and other nutritious foods. If you have to go a little out of your way to get a food, you'll have more time to consider why you might be overeating it. Work through the issue; don't ignore it.

## SOLUTION

### CONQUER AN ALL-OR-NOTHING MINDSET

"I am all-or-nothing when it comes to dieting." I hear this all the time from clients. It's often accompanied by a pattern of starting off the day "great" and, like clockwork, it unravels by the evening. Self-talk can often sound like "Well, I was really good all day, so I deserve this" or "Well, I already blew my diet, so I might as well keep going." Either way, the all-or-nothing attitude is not a permanent personality trait; it's a product of dieting and a dysfunctional relationship with food. Here are some strategies to break free of this detrimental mindset and find a middle ground:

- **Lower your expectations.** Stop expecting perfection. Aim for the 80/20 approach instead: Plan to eat nutritiously and balanced 80 percent of the time, leaving 20 percent for the unplanned. Eat what your body *needs* 80 percent of the time and eat what your mind *craves* the rest of the time.
- **Allow flexibility.** Accept that your body does not burn the same amount of energy every day, so you cannot expect to eat the same way every day and feel satisfied.
- **Stop labeling foods.** If you eat a "bad" food, you will feel bad, and that reinforces other behaviors that make you feel even worse. You may believe eating the "bad" food gives you license to just keep going. Instead, categorize foods as more nutritious or healthier versus less nutritious or less healthy.
- **Figure out why.** Ruminating over *what* already happened is not productive. Focus on *why* it happened instead. Use the experience as a lesson and move on with positive intentions.
- **Give yourself a pass.** If you ate something you regret, that is okay! One meal, or one day of eating, will not destroy your future.

Finding this balance can be challenging. Be patient with yourself as you improve.

**The Obsessive Eater**

Obsessive Eaters are the most at risk of developing an eating disorder (if one doesn't already exist). In addition, any of the other three archetypes can spiral into an Obsessive Eater if left untreated. These eaters constantly worry about food and how it affects weight or health. Controlling and manipulating food may be a coping mechanism for life stressors or disappointments.

### CHARACTERISTIC BEHAVIORS
- Fear of weight gain and a struggle with body dysmorphia (fixating on flaws)
- Restricting intake to the point that it affects energy, mood, concentration, and (for women) ovulation
- Resorting to compensatory behavior like exercising or restriction after overeating
- Alternating between restriction and overeating or binge-eating
- Using devices to obsessively track weight, food portions, and calorie intake

### THE PITFALLS OF THE OBSESSIVE EATER
- An eating disorder diagnosis
- Anxiety and distress around mealtimes
- Health complications such as hair loss, nutritional deficiencies, hormonal imbalances (infertility), bone and muscle loss, metabolic decline, and in severe cases, death

Tips to remedy these issues include seeking professional help, especially to release the urge to control through scales and apps.

## SOLUTION

### QUIET THE NOISE

There is often a lot of noise inside the mind of an Obsessive Eater. The noise is a combination of different voices dictating food choices, second-guessing decisions, and implanting guilt and shame. The more you let this noise control your every move, the harder it will be to keep it quiet. Find the healthier voice that has been buried down deep—the voice that drives you to nourish yourself, eat food whenever you need to, and form a healthier relationship with food.

## SOLUTION

### SEEK PROFESSIONAL HELP

Professional help is mandatory. Private treatment through a multidisciplinary approach, including a licensed therapist, dietitian, and primary care doctor, is step one. A therapist can help unpack psychological trauma or childhood experiences that may have increased the risk of eating disorders. A dietitian will ensure balanced eating and offer support to eat a sufficient, varied diet.

The Core Three Plan prioritizes balanced eating in a nonrestrictive and personalized way. However, it can still be triggering for those with very serious unresolved food relationship issues. If you fall under this archetype, I strongly advise that you seek professional help. This book is not a substitute for medical advice and is not intended to diagnose or treat anyone with a serious medical issue.

## SOLUTION

### RELINQUISH CONTROL

Put away control methods and devices such as scales, and delete apps that are encouraging obsessive behaviors. The more you try to control, the less in control you'll be. Learning how to trust and appreciate your body can also help to alleviate the need to supervise every single bite of food. Stop diets that are calorie-restrictive or eliminate food groups; they will further unhealthy food views.

A healthy relationship with food is one that allows for freedom from guilt and freedom of choice. It means eating in a balanced way and including a variety of foods that you both *want* and *need*. Being flexible, not rigid, is crucial to succeed. Staying aware of your habits and practicing the solutions you read in this chapter will help you heal your relationship with food and/or prevent distorted eating.

The more you continue to work on this relationship by improving your outlook, attitudes, and behaviors around eating, the easier it will become. Aim for progress, not perfection. Now that you've done some reflection and introspection on your personal attitudes toward eating, let's move into Part Two, which introduces the fundamentals of the Core Three Plan.

# 2 THE BASICS OF THE PLAN

# CHAPTER 3

# The Core Three Way of Eating

deally, we would not need a nutrition plan to figure out how to eat to meet our bodies' needs and find food freedom. We would simply rely on intuition and our own natural-born hunger and fullness cues. The reality is that there are many circumstances, including stress, schedules, resources, finances, medical issues, and mental health, that interfere with our ability to listen and respond to these innate cues. At some point in the future, as you work through the steps of securing your food-and-body connection, you will overcome some of these obstacles. For now, use these guidelines in the Core Three Healthy Eating Plan as your training wheels until you find your own natural balance to eat more freely.

In this chapter, you will learn the Core Three Healthy Eating Plan guidelines and how to follow and structure the plan to fit your needs. You will also see how you can continue to adjust the plan as you improve your relationship with food and your body. Personalization is key, so you will receive clear instructions on how to adjust portions to match your weight, sex at birth, and activity level. This chapter also covers meal timing and hydration. I will also explain why the Core Three does not require calorie counting and why balanced, inclusive eating is the cornerstone to eating healthier and weighing "happy."

## An Introduction to the Core Three Healthy Eating Plan

The premise of the Core Three is simple: Eat a strategic balance of macronutrients that will support health and fuel your body. It employs the number three throughout to make it easy to remember. Here are the key guidelines:

- Start with *three* servings of carbohydrates, with more added if needed based on your individual factors (explained later).
  - Try to include at least one serving of fruit in your total carbs for the day.
  - Exchange 1–2 carbs for a treat or discretionary snack like wine, chocolate, ice cream, or chips, if desired. We call these "flexible carbs," and I will explain them more later.
- Eat a minimum of *three* servings of lean proteins, with more added if needed based on your individual factors.
- Include a variety of lean animal- and plant-based proteins from the Core Three list. (Additional instructions will be provided for vegan or vegetarian diets.)
- Consume a minimum of *three* servings of anti-inflammatory fats, with more added if needed based on your individual factors.

- Focus on consuming monounsaturated fats and certain polyunsaturated fats from the tables provided in Chapter 6.
- Incorporate *three* servings of non-starchy veggies or more per day.
- Aim to include the *three* essential food groups at each meal as often as possible for optimal nutrient absorption, blood glucose control, and satiety.
- Aim for a minimum of 25 grams of fiber per day. The fiber content of foods is included in all of your Core Three food tables (provided in Chapters 4–7).
- Exercise moderately *three* hours per week.
- Aim to drink up to *three* liters of water per day (about 100 ounces).
- Keep food journals for a minimum of *three* weeks and preferably for at least *three* months.
- Give yourself *three* weeks to fairly track progress before making any adjustments.

The Core Three Healthy Eating Plan is not a one-size-fits-all plan—it is meant to be personalized and made your own. It is a forever formula that is intended to enable you to treat your body as an ally. Wellness is a skill, and this plan helps you practice prioritizing a healthy relationship with food to promote healthy eating and long-term behavioral change.

## Core Three Meal Structure

Remember, on the Core Three, the number three is your guide. At *each* meal, aim to include all *three* macronutrients—although that may not happen at every meal. Consume an appropriate portion of carbs, fats, and proteins at *each* meal. Non-starchy veggies can be enjoyed more liberally. Eventually, lean proteins and anti-inflammatory fats can also be enjoyed ad libitum as you practice listening and responding to your innate cues.

Although I set a minimum portion for each food group, it is unrealistic and unscientific to assume that everyone should eat the same amount of carbs, proteins, and fats per day, regardless of activity level, body size, and sex. That's why you will learn, in the following sections, how to customize and personalize this plan to better meet your nutritional needs and promote healthy weight loss. The Core Three formula provides the recommended daily servings to jump-start your healthy weight loss journey. As you become more familiar with balanced eating and notice sufficient weight loss—around the 3-month mark—you can gradually liberalize the plan by only portioning out carbs, and not proteins or fats, to exercise more food freedom. That doesn't mean you will stop achieving your weight loss goals. It is just an appropriate time to start practicing letting your body guide your food choices. Eventually listening to your body will take precedence over any plan, and you will not need to keep track of servings as carefully.

### How Many Servings of Carbs Do You Need?

The 2020–2025 Dietary Guidelines for Americans recommend that you consume around 45–65 percent of your total calories from carbohydrates. The Core Three Plan understands this amount is often too high for most individuals who wish to find their happiest weight. For that reason, you'll be eating closer to 35 percent of your total calories per day from carbohydrates. To achieve that, start with a minimum of three servings per day. Then (if you do not know your exact weight, select an approximate range):

- Add one serving if you were assigned male at birth (total of 4).
- Add one additional serving if you weigh 150 pounds or more (total of 4 for female; 5 for male).
- Add one additional serving if you weigh 200 pounds or more (total of 5 for female; 6 for male).
- Add one additional serving if you weigh more than 250 pounds (total of 6 for female; 7 for male).

Calculate the number of servings you need based on your weight and write that number here: _____ servings. This is your personalized portion and the number of servings you are to consume each day. Aim to evenly divide your portion among three meals throughout your day.

### How the Core Three Formula Was Created

The guide considers several factors, including weight. That's because the more you weigh, the more food your body may need. Think about it this way: It is easier to walk up a flight of stairs empty-armed than it is with a thirty-pound stack of books. The latter requires more energy and effort to reach the top. That's how it works when you have more body mass. Though weight is not always the best marker of overall health, we will use your current weight to guide your meal structure as you get started.

We will discuss exercise recommendations in Chapter 8, but if you exercise moderately to intensely more than 3 hours per week, add one additional serving of carbs for the day. If you have any special medical conditions or hormonal imbalances or you're breastfeeding, you may need to further adjust the serving size up or down. If you fall into those categories, review these special conditions in Chapter 10 before beginning the program.

### WHAT A CORE THREE CARBOHYDRATE SERVING LOOKS LIKE

Because you're tracking your carbohydrate intake, it's important to clearly define a carbohydrate serving size on the Core Three. *One carbohydrate serving is equivalent to about 20 grams of net carbs and an average of 100 calories.* Chapter 4 will explain carbohydrates in greater detail and provide lists of carbohydrate foods to choose. Smaller amounts of carbohydrates are also present in other Core Three macro foods such as certain proteins and fats, as well as non-starchy veggies. We do not refer to these food groups as "carbohydrates" on this plan. In the Core Three Healthy Eating Plan, foods are categorized based on the majority source of their calories. Non-starchy vegetables, discussed in Chapter 7, provide bulk and energizing nutrients like fiber and antioxidants.

If you are eating more than three servings of carbohydrates per day, you can double up servings at certain meals (like having two slices of bread instead of one), incorporate carbs as a snack in between meals (like an apple or crackers), or potentially exchange one for a satisfying treat. Keep your carbohydrates spaced out evenly to support healthy energy, digestion, and metabolism.

### Calculating Carb Counts Using Nutritional Labels

You'll find a wide variety of foods and their Core Three carb servings listed in Chapter 4, but you will likely also want to eat foods not listed. Here is a formula to determine how many Core Three carb servings are in any product you pick up at the store.

Let's look at a nutrition label from the FDA together:

**Nutrition Facts**

8 servings per container

Serving size 2/3 cup (55g)

Amount per serving

**Calories** 230

% Daily Value*

| | |
|---|---|
| **Total Fat** 8g | **10%** |
| Saturated Fat 1g | **5%** |
| *Trans* Fat 0g | |
| **Cholesterol** 0mg | **0%** |
| **Sodium** 160mg | **7%** |
| **Total Carbohydrate** 37g | **13%** |
| Dietary Fiber 4g | **14%** |
| Total Sugars 12g | |
| Includes 10g Added Sugars | **20%** |
| **Protein** 3g | |
| Vitamin D 2mcg | 10% |
| Calcium 260mg | 20% |
| Iron 8mg | 45% |
| Potassium 235mg | 6% |

* The % Daily Value (DV) tells you how much a nutrient in a serving of food contributes to a daily diet. 2,000 calories a day is used for general nutrition advice.

First, subtract the "dietary fiber" (in this case, 4 grams) from "total carbohydrates" (37 grams) to get the net grams of carbohydrates (33 grams). This food has 33 grams of NET carbs per ⅔-cup serving. How many "carbs" is this in the Core Three Plan?

- 10–15 grams of NET carbs ~ ½ carb serving

- 16–25 grams of NET carbs ~ 1 carb serving
- 26–35 grams of NET carbs ~ 1½ carb servings
- 36–45 grams of NET carbs ~ 2 carb servings

Therefore, if you ate one serving of this food as designated on the label (⅔ cup), you would be consuming 1½ Core Three carbs. If you wanted this food to count toward only one of your three daily carbs, you could reduce the portion size. Any food product serving that has less than 10 grams of net carbs is negligible and does not count as a carb serving.

**What Are Net Carbs?**

Net carbs are what remains after subtracting the nondigestible carbs, such as total fiber and sugar alcohols. For example, if a food has 30 grams of carbohydrates per serving and 10 grams of fiber, the total net carbs is 20 grams. You digest and absorb only 20 grams of carbohydrates; the rest continues down your gastrointestinal highway. Since fiber is predominantly nondigestible, you do not count it when carb-tracking, especially when trying to manage blood sugars to facilitate weight loss. All the more reason to fill up on fiber! However, this may depend on the person. Those who need to monitor blood glucose levels more closely and are more insulin resistant or carb-sensitive may still react to higher-carbohydrate foods despite the total number of "net carbs." Besides fiber, sugar alcohols are also nondigestible carbohydrates that can be subtracted from "net carbs."

**SUGAR ALCOHOLS**

Sugar alcohols do not actually contain alcohol. They are naturally occurring compounds found in some fruits and veggies, but they can also be manufactured. Sugar alcohols are often added to foods, such as sugar-free candy, ice cream, chewing gum, and protein bars, as a lower-sugar sweetener. They will increase blood glucose levels less than traditional sugar does. Hence, they are often subtracted from total carbs.

It is common for people to rely on these lower-calorie and lower-sugar options to prevent weight gain. However, when consumed in large quantities, they can have a laxative effect. Either way, always ask yourself, "Is this even enjoyable? If I just ate the original version of chocolate, ice cream, or candy, would I feel more satisfied and possibly eat less?"

**How Many Servings of Lean Protein Do You Need?**

Controversy surrounds recommended protein amounts, and many experts, including myself, believe established requirements fall short. The Dietary Guidelines for Americans recommend 10–35 percent of your calories come from protein. The Core Three incorporates the higher end, or 25–35 percent of total calories per day, to support lean muscle preservation and help keep you satisfied.

### Does Excess Protein Lead to Bulking Up?

Despite popular belief, eating more protein will not change your body type. While amino acids derived from protein assist with muscle repair, recovery, and growth, this is not a limitless process. We can typically utilize only around 30 grams of protein at one sitting, depending on various factors like activity level, lean body mass, and sex. After that, excess protein is burned or stored as fuel, and any unused amino acids are excreted through urine. Manufacturing muscles usually requires higher amounts of total calories, a specific exercise regimen, and genetics. For example, women are not genetically inclined to build muscle as easily as men, even with a heavy weightlifting routine, mainly due to differences in sex hormones like testosterone.

Protein consumption also matters based on other factors:

- **Age:** At around age forty, you start to lose more muscle through a process called sarcopenia. Increasing protein can help mitigate natural muscle atrophy.
- **Sex:** If you were assigned male at birth, your body may require more protein to preserve naturally higher muscle mass.

- **Diet:** Vegetarians and vegans who consume limited or no animal protein sources need to compensate with additional plant protein to offset the dietary exclusion.
- **Activity:** The more physically active you are, the greater your energy and protein demands will be. If you exercise more than 3 hours per week, chances are you can benefit from increased protein consumption.

To find your ideal amount, refer to the same formula that you used to determine carb servings—your protein servings will ultimately match your carb servings. Calculate the number of servings you need based on your weight and write that number here: _____ servings. This is your personalized portion and the number of servings you should aim for each day. Aim to evenly divide your portion among three meals throughout your day.

### WHAT A CORE THREE LEAN PROTEIN SERVING LOOKS LIKE

Again, it's important to clearly define a lean protein serving size on the Core Three. *One protein serving is equivalent to an average of 20 grams of protein and a range of 100–150 calories.*

To calculate protein servings using nutrition labels, you can use the following reference:

- 8–14 grams of protein: ½ protein serving
- 15–25 grams of protein: 1 protein serving
- 26–35 grams of protein: 1½ protein servings
- 36–45 grams of protein: 2 protein servings

If a product has less than 8 grams of protein, it does not need to count toward your protein servings.

### How Many Servings of Anti-Inflammatory Fats Do You Need?

The Dietary Guidelines for Americans recommend that up to 35 percent of your total daily calories come from fat, which aligns with the Core Three Plan. Refer to the same formula that you used to determine carb servings—your fat servings will ultimately match your carb and protein servings. Calculate the number of servings you need based on your weight and write that number here: _____ servings. This is your personalized portion and the number of servings you should aim for each day. Aim to evenly divide your portion among three meals throughout your day.

## WHAT A CORE THREE ANTI-INFLAMMATORY FAT SERVING LOOKS LIKE

An anti-inflammatory fat serving size on the Core Three *is equivalent to about 10 grams of fat and an average of 100 calories.*

To calculate fat servings using nutrition labels, you can use the following reference:

- 5–7 grams of fat: ½ fat serving
- 8–12 grams of fat: 1 fat serving
- 13–16 grams of fat: 1½ fat servings
- 17–22 grams of fat: 2 fat servings

If a product has less than 5 grams of fat, it does not need to count toward your fat servings.

### Food Freedom and Weight Maintenance

If your goals are more about finding food freedom and maintaining your current healthy, happy weight, then it may be best to avoid counting altogether as it can distract you from practicing listening to your body. In that case, simply focus on eating a variety of high-fiber carbs, lean proteins, and anti-inflammatory fats. It may still help to aim to include all three at every meal as much as possible. Review Chapters 1 and 2 to work on improving your relationship with food and your body. I will explain how to maintain weight after weight loss in Chapter 11.

## Meal Timing

Timing and frequency of eating can have an impact on your appetite and energy. Ideally, you will listen to your body to determine when it's time to eat. Using hunger cues and practicing rating your hunger on a scale of 1–10 (where 1 is uncomfortably full and 10 is ravenous) to guide you is the first step. Hunger is a physiological response from your brain when it senses your stomach is empty. Yet, other factors can interfere with your ability to gauge true hunger. Emotions (like stress or boredom), distractions, triggers, environmental factors, and lack of access to food (or, conversely, consuming too much food) can make it difficult to accurately detect hunger.

Establishing an eating routine makes a difference in preventing overeating or undereating. Eating too frequently will likely lead to overeating, but skipping meals can backfire as well. Regular nourishment prevents blood sugar crashes and strong cravings and encourages balanced food choices. Longer pauses in eating also create more hunger. The hungrier you are, the harder it is to think clearly about what you should put into your body. We also tend to eat faster when we wait too long to eat.

Typically, true biological hunger occurs every 3–5 hours throughout the day, depending on the size of your prior meal. Try to follow this timing when planning your meals for the day. If you eat breakfast at 9:00 a.m., try not wait longer than 2:00 p.m. before putting some combo of high-fiber carb, lean protein, and anti-inflammatory fat into your system.

Of course, if you are not a breakfast person or have a very long day that requires multiple snacks to get by, you can make adjustments. As long as you're not intentionally skipping or prolonging meals or, by contrast, eating all day regardless of physiological hunger, the times you eat should fit into your lifestyle.

## Arranging Your Macronutrient Portions Throughout the Day

In addition to considering the timing of your meals, think about how you are spreading out your food portions over the day. Though you are aiming to incorporate carbohydrates, lean proteins, and anti-inflammatory fats at each meal, you have flexibility to reorder these macros as you prefer. Non-starchy veggies can also be eaten at any point in the day, whether it's with a meal or between meals—as long

### What about Intermittent Fasting?

Intermittent fasting (IF) has created a buzz in recent years, although this restrained eating pattern began in the early 1900s. There are several types of IF, but the most popular approach is the 16:8 method, which involves eating only within an 8-hour period of the day, such as from 12:00 to 8:00 p.m. or 8:00 a.m. to 4:00 p.m. Other methods include fasting for an entire day a couple days per week. While the guidelines are flexible, the overarching idea is the same: Avoid eating for an extended time to promote insulin reduction and fat-burning. Weight loss and improvements in energy, digestion, blood sugars, and cholesterol may also occur. Current research shows both favorable and unfavorable outcomes. Some studies support these benefits, while other studies show few benefits. Issues present when you take meal-dependent medications, enjoy regular exercise that requires sufficient pre- and post-workout fuel, or have a history of disordered eating. Those who skip breakfast to adhere to fasting guidelines may also find they are thinking about food more throughout the day, which can lead to overeating. For these reasons, the Core Three philosophy is to listen to your body first and not place more restrictions around eating than necessary. You don't need to fast to feel your healthiest.

If you still want to introduce the concept of fasting, my recommendation is a 12-hour fast between your last meal of the day and your first meal of the next day. This is enough to acquire some of the perceived benefits without affecting your relationship with food. So, if you normally eat breakfast around 7:30 a.m., aim to complete your final meal by 7:30 p.m. the night before. Importantly, don't deprive yourself or fight against the basic human need for food.

as there are a minimum of three servings per day. For example, if your personalized counts are 3 carbs, 3 proteins, and 3 fats, you could do the following:

- Breakfast: 1 carb, 1 protein
- Lunch: 1 carb, 1 protein, 1 fat, 2 non-starchy veggies
- Snack: 1 carb, 1 fat
- Dinner: 1 protein, 1 fat, 2 non-starchy veggies

In this case, there is not a carb, protein, and fat at every meal, but it is evenly distributed enough to fit the plan.

Another example of how you could arrange your plan if your counts are 4 carbs, 4 proteins, and 4 fats is as follows:

- Breakfast: 1 protein, 1 fat, 1 non-starchy veggie
- Lunch: 2 carbs, 1 protein, 1 fat
- Snack: 1 carb, 1 fat
- Dinner: 1 carb, 2 proteins, 1 fat, 2 non-starchy veggies

Here you will see that some meals don't contain all three macros, but again, it is distributed evenly enough to support the premise of the plan.

Ideally, you will still aim to arrange your macros in a way that maintains balance, but you must be flexible with how that plays out from day to day.

## Hydration and Health

Hydration is an essential part of Core Three principles. About 60 percent of your body is made of water. Water helps with nutrient absorption and body temperature regulation, lubricates joints and organs, and protects heart function. Filling up on fluids also promotes adequate energy, cognition, and bowel movement, as well as appetite regularity. A 2008 study published in the journal *Obesity* that was conducted on 173 overweight women, ages 25–50, discovered a positive correlation between drinking more water and significant body fat loss over time. Water also helps push the high-fiber foods you'll be eating through your system, keeps you energized, and flushes out toxins.

A common misconception is that drinking water increases water retention and bloat, making you feel uncomfortable or leading you to believe you've gained weight. It actually does the opposite: It fights against water retention and swelling. The higher your water intake, the less your body feels pressured to retain.

### How Much Water Should I Drink?

One way to determine your water needs is to observe the color of your urine. The lighter the color, the more hydrated you are. But not everyone can rely on this method or remember to constantly look down before flushing. For that reason, it is simpler and safer to aim for 2–3 liters of unsweetened water per day (about eight to twelve 8-ounce glasses or 70–100 ounces) for proper hydration. You may need the higher end of the range if you are more active, are a heavy sweater, or weigh over 200 pounds. If this feels like a daunting task, start slowly by gradually adding in at least one 8-ounce glass of water with, or before, every meal and snack. If you're not a fan of plain $H_2O$, there are natural ways to spruce up your beverages. Infusing water with fresh fruit (like orange or lime slices), mint leaves, or cucumber can make it more appealing. You can also rotate in sparkling water and seltzer.

## How Soon Will I See Results?

First you will *feel* the results of the Core Three Eating Plan, and then you will *see* them. You will notice improvements in energy, digestion, mood, and sleep as soon as you begin to make changes toward a more balanced diet along with healthy behavior modifications. When you start focusing on your relationship with food and your body by understanding what type of eater you are and areas you need to work on, you will discover a novel experience never felt with any other diet plan. The Core Three is about improving your relationship with food, so it's not just about seeing the number on the scale, or your clothing size, go down.

If weight loss is what you're after and your relationship with food is solid, or it's something you have been working on, then know that progress is rarely linear. Don't expect to see instant results every single week. Practice patience and remain positive. First, you will feel improvements in the way your clothes are fitting and your energy levels are improving. Healthy weight loss is around 1–2 pounds per week. After that, you might notice consistent weight loss, but if not, that doesn't mean it's not working. Don't get discouraged. Everyone is different, and instead of getting too caught up in the number on the scale, pay attention to those other improvements in your life and how you are feeling overall. We will specifically discuss how to measure progress in Chapter 11, but if it has been several weeks and you're still stalled, there will be more instructions on how to accelerate the plan in Chapter 9. Remember, if you are trying to find your happiest weight, the longer it takes to come off, the longer it stays off.

## Calories Power Your Body

A calorie is a unit of energy, and weight changes can certainly be influenced by *calories in versus calories out*—or how many calories you consume compared with how many you burn. While calorie-counting is not a major focus on this plan, a calorie deficit is warranted to produce weight loss; however, determining your calorie threshold for weight loss is not so simple. The number of calories you expend in a day is not only based on variable factors including exercise and physical activity. A large percentage, or up to 75 percent, of our daily calorie expenditure comes from our resting metabolic rate (RMR). A RMR refers to how much energy your body uses during rest for involuntary, vital actions such as your heart beating, breathing, and the digestive process. It may seem as though your RMR is a relatively fixed figure, but it can fluctuate based on changes in exercise, diet, age, medications, and medical conditions. For that reason, it is almost impossible to pinpoint the exact number of calories you burn every day, especially for a prolonged time period. Therefore, it is impossible to know the exact number of calories to consume to create a calorie deficit.

While we are on the topic, the other reason we don't fixate on calories is because not all calories are digested and metabolized the same way. The calories in a soft drink will not offer the same quality of energy as a bowl of fresh fruit. The more nutritious your calories are, the more staying power and energy they will provide; you will feel fuller longer, which will make it easier to eat what your body needs without overeating. Another common mistake my clients make is avoiding high-calorie foods like almond butter, avocado, and olive oil. Instead, they will choose lower-calorie options such as

rice cakes, diet sodas, and hundred-calorie packs of cookies. Avocados might have more calories than many other foods, but think about what you're getting with those calories.

The final explanation why calorie-counting is not an encouraged long-term practice is because doing so distracts you from truly listening to your body. If you are primarily focused on the calorie price tag, you are probably not paying attention to your innate hunger and fullness cues. You can't truly listen to your body when you are distracted by diligently counting your calories. You don't need to micromanage every calorie you consume for weight loss—your body can handle it!

If you have always been calorie-conscious and are not ready to say goodbye to keeping track, or you are simply wondering exactly how much you'll be eating on this plan, there is a strategic range. The minimum, core plan comes out to roughly 1,200 calories per day when you're including every recommended food group—carbs, proteins, fats, and non-starchy veggies. The next tier, or 4:4:4 (carbs:proteins:fats), is approximately 1,500 calories per day, and 5:5:5 is around 1,800 calories per day. Essentially, it goes up in increments of 300 calories. Some days, your total daily calories may clock in a little lower than this estimate and other days your totals may clock in a little higher. That is okay; however, if you are following the 3:3:3 plan and notice you have dipped far below 1,200 calories, then it is important to adjust. It could be because your portions are smaller than what it is recommend in the Core Three food charts. Finally, it could also be a discrepancy in the calorie-counting app or system you're using.

If your goal is weight loss, you may have learned it's best to keep calories as low as possible. The reality is that eating too few calories can be just as detrimental for weight loss as eating too many. Not only does undereating increase risk of nutrient deficiencies that may affect bone density, hormonal balance (fertility), digestion (constipation), and even mood, but it can also slow metabolism. Ultimately, if you want to stoke your metabolic fire, you need to eat a sufficient number of calories. The Core Three Healthy Eating Plan will assure you are properly nourished.

## Understanding Macronutrients

Carbohydrates, proteins, and fats are the three major *macronutrients*, or nutrients that are required in larger amounts to support basic physiological functions. Each macro has an important role:

- Carbohydrates are our premier source of energy.
- Proteins provide the building blocks for repair.
- Fats support cell growth, as well as hormonal balance.

They also work synergistically to maximize absorption, metabolism, and energy. For example, carbs help protein get to your muscles, especially post-exercise. Fats help slow the breakdown of carbs, and they also help your body absorb fat-soluble nutrients found in proteins and carbohydrates.

You can identify any food on your plate as a carbohydrate, protein, or fat. Some foods contain only one macronutrient, but most foods contain a mixture of two, or even all three, of these macronutrients. For example:

- Protein-rich foods like salmon and eggs also contain fats.
- Fat-rich foods like nuts also contain protein and even some carbs.
- Carb-rich foods like quinoa and black beans also contain protein.

Even though these overlaps are common, on the Core Three Healthy Eating Plan, foods are categorized based on the majority source of their calories. For example, a ⅔-cup serving of black beans has about 26 grams of carbohydrates and 9 grams of protein; therefore, the Core Three categorizes black beans as a carb. Nuts are another example. Many people rely on nuts as a protein source or assume they are a high-protein food. While they are certainly a *good* source of protein, as well as other nutrients like fiber, iron, magnesium, and antioxidants, they have twice as much fat as they do protein. A 1-ounce serving of almonds has almost 14 grams of fat and just under 6 grams of protein. No matter how they're combined, our bodies rely on these core macronutrients for energy, repair, growth, and maintenance—and that's why they are essential on the Core Three Healthy Eating Plan.

We will take a closer look at all three macronutrients in the subsequent chapters and learn how to eat healthfully and for weight management.

The Core Three way of eating was created to empower you to make the necessary changes to feel your best. It's not just about weight loss and, in fact, for some of you, it shouldn't be about that at all. Although you just received a quick overview of why the three macronutrients are essential for your overall health, in the next three chapters, we'll drill down and explore each one in more depth. This is also where you will receive explicit food charts to guide you toward making the best choices for your body.

CHAPTER 4

# High-Fiber Carbohydrates

From what I have observed, the war against carbs has spiraled out of control. Foods like bread, pasta, and cereal are notorious for being on the "do not eat" list on most diet plans. While studies do show that reducing carbs can help with weight loss, you still *need* to eat carbs to sustain any weight loss diet. Why? Because carbs add variety and vital nutrients to your diet that promote healthy energy levels. They make meals more satisfying and enjoyable. Cutting out carbs, or any major food groups, not only unravels your relationship with food but also contributes to intense cravings. Restricting carbs can also result in the loss of lean muscle mass that impacts your body composition. Most importantly, they are our primary source of energy—our battery pack. They supply glucose to our bodies, which is like gasoline for a car. That's why carbohydrates—an essential macronutrient—are not only allowed but *encouraged* from day one of the Core Three Healthy Eating Plan.

Carbohydrates, which predominantly come in the form of whole grains, legumes, fruits, and vegetables, are also the most abundant source of antioxidants, critical vitamins, and digestion-regulating fiber (which can support your metabolism). Not all carbohydrates are digested, absorbed, and metabolized the same way, however. Focusing on specific types of carbohydrates can make the difference when it comes to healthy energy and weight management.

In this chapter, you will learn why high-fiber carbohydrates are highlighted on the Core Three, what carbohydrates are, and how they influence weight and health. We will dive into why cutting out carbohydrates is not the answer and why they are not all created equally—digestion rate makes a difference. Fiber is a core component of the Core Three Plan, and I will explain why that's a primary reason you need to include carbs for healthy weight loss. We will also discuss the controversies behind sugar and why completely banning sugar from your diet is not the answer either. This chapter also contains the Core Three carbohydrate tables, which include portion sizes and fiber content for specific types of high-fiber carbs, as well as some satisfying low-carb alternatives.

# What Are Carbohydrates?

Carbohydrates are an essential macronutrient predominantly found in grains, fruits, starchy veggies, dairy, and sweet-tasting foods. They offer the most readily available source of energy compared to proteins and fats. Carbohydrates are 4 calories per gram, which means a typical slice of wheat bread with 20 grams of carbohydrates is about 80 calories.

## How Carbs Affect Weight

Although carbohydrates can contribute to weight gain, it does not happen overnight and depends on a confluence of factors like types and quantities of carbs consumed, individual activity level, metabolism, stress, sleep, and insulin sensitivity. Let's discuss how carbs are used and stored to gain a better understanding of the process.

### THE SCIENCE OF CARBS

After consumption, all carbs eventually get broken down into a simple sugar, or monosaccharide, called glucose. Whether you're enjoying a fruit salad or spinning your fork into a bowl of spaghetti, glucose is the end result after digestion and absorption. Glucose is like gasoline to a car—it keeps us moving and functioning. It travels through your bloodstream, signaling your brain to release insulin hormone from your pancreas. Insulin's primary function is to transport this glucose (or sugar) to your cells for energy use or storage.

### Complex vs. Simple Carbs

Carbs can be categorized as complex or simple depending upon their molecular structure; however, those categories can be a little confusing when it comes to how nutritious they are and how quickly they are digested. You might think that all "complex" carbs contain more nutrients than "simple" carbs, but that's not always the case. Most complex carbs, including whole grains, veggies, and beans, *are* nutritious and digested more slowly. Refined flours such as white flour and white rice are also considered complex but are digested more quickly and with less nutritional value. On the other hand, most simple carbs, also referred to as added sugars—refined sugar, syrups, and honey—are digested rapidly. Nutrient-dense fruit contains a simple carb, or natural sugar (fructose), but is digested slower than other simple carbs.

For that reason, it is more productive to focus on how carbohydrates are digested and how nutritious they are rather than on whether they are complex or simple. Please see the "Slower- vs. Faster-Digesting Carbs" section later in this chapter for more information.

Your body does not like to waste any energy. As insulin funnels glucose to your cells, whatever is not used for energy gets stored as glycogen in your muscle and liver—it does not immediately get stored as fat. Only after these stores are filled does your body store excess glucose as body fat.

Studies also show that insulin can influence appetite and directly prevent fat loss. After we eat a meal, insulin levels rise. The more quick-digesting carbs you eat, the higher they will go. That insulin sends a message to your brain: "We have enough fuel coming in as food—there is no need to burn, or utilize, fat stores for fuel." Therefore, the more quick-digesting carbs you consume, the higher the resulting levels of blood sugars, then insulin levels, and finally, the accumulation of body fat will be. Thus, eating slower-digesting carbs in combination with other macronutrients like lean proteins and anti-inflammatory fats is the winning ticket for weight management.

**THE SATISFACTION THAT CARBS OFFER**

It may seem like carbs are the foods to blame for all your weight woes. However, cutting out too many carbs can be just as detrimental to your weight loss progress as eating too many. Why?

Carbohydrates contribute a ton of satisfaction to meals. What would a sandwich be without bread, and what would cereal taste like without the actual cereal? You don't need to find out. Without that satisfaction factor, cravings and urges for starchier, sugary foods can skyrocket.

Carbohydrates are also the leading source of fiber, which is a crucial ingredient in the Core Three success formula.

This is important because high-fiber carbs fight against constipation and bloat that can stall weight loss progress and, more importantly, make you feel uncomfortable. We will discuss more on fiber later in this chapter to learn additional reasons it can promote healthy weight loss.

### Blame the Weight Gain on the Water, Not the Carbs

If you feel like you instantly gain weight whenever you even look at a bowl of pasta, water might partly be the culprit. When glucose is stored as glycogen, it latches on to a water molecule. A 2015 randomized controlled trial in the *European Journal of Applied Physiology* clarifies that "each gram of glycogen is stored with at least 3 grams of water, although higher ratios are possible." This may explain why some people may feel heavier and more bloated and possibly see an immediate uptick on the scale after eating a higher-carb meal. There could be other reasons for these uncomfortable symptoms and water weight in general, but carbs do increase water retention in the body, and it has nothing to do with body fat.

When your body isn't receiving enough carb-derived energy, it can retaliate. How so? It doesn't only burn fat, but it can also burn protein in your muscle. Carbs also facilitate muscle growth, so depriving your body of carbs can also block lean-muscle building. Eating enough protein can help prevent this, but not everyone does that! We will talk more about proteins in the next chapter. For these reasons, you need carbohydrates, and although they are portioned on this plan, they are still absolutely encouraged.

### Slower- vs. Faster-Digesting Carbs

You can think of carbs in two categories—slower-digesting and faster-digesting. Slower-digesting carbs are typically higher in fiber, which slows down the rate of digestion. As a result, you end up feeling fuller and have more stable blood sugars and insulin levels, which can help modulate appetite and encourage fat-burning. That's why slower-digesting carbs are beneficial, even for weight loss. Here are some common carbs and whether they are slow- or fast-digesting:

**SLOWER-DIGESTING CARBS**
- Whole grains (oats, quinoa, whole wheat, sprouted whole grains, teff)
- Sweet potatoes
- Beans/lentils
- Fruits
- Dairy

**FASTER-DIGESTING CARBS**
- Refined flours like white flour
- White rice
- Refined sugar
- Syrups
- Honey

Keep in mind that the rate at which some of these foods are digested also depends on what they are eaten with. Let's discuss more about slower- and faster-digesting carbs.

## What Makes a Carb Slower-Digesting?

The best way to determine the rate at which you digest, or break down, specific carbohydrates is to check your individual blood sugar and insulin levels. Since most of us don't have access to this kind of test on a regular basis, there is an easier method to predict how your body will respond to certain foods—namely, determining its fiber content. Fiber is a type of carbohydrate that is naturally found in plant-based foods such as fruits, veggies, beans, whole grains, nuts, and seeds.

### The Importance of Fiber

Generally, the more fiber the carbohydrate contains, the longer it may take to break down and digest in your digestive tract. Any carbohydrate that has 5 grams of fiber or more is considered a "high-fiber" food. Why does fiber influence digestion rate? Because it is mostly a nondigestible carbohydrate that absorbs water and expands as it moves through your gastrointestinal system. This process also leads to numerous other benefits beyond slowing down carb digestion:

- Fiber expands in your stomach, making you feel more satisfied for a sustained period of time, improving blood sugar regulation, and suppressing insulin levels. Therefore, fiber can also help prevent type 2 diabetes.
- Fiber-filled foods regulate bowel movements, fighting constipation.
- Fiber feeds healthy gut bacteria through the production of short-chain fatty acids, allowing them to flourish to support higher metabolism levels.
- Fiber has been linked to improved blood pressure and cholesterol levels, lowering the risk factors for heart disease.

### Consuming Excess Fiber

While your body can handle more than 25 grams of fiber, excessive amounts—over 50–60 grams—can produce digestive issues like gas and bloating. Symptoms like these will depend upon the type of fiber eaten in addition to other factors. Consuming a variety of fibers, adding them in gradually if you're not used to consuming much, and drinking plenty of water can prevent digestive distress.

Unfortunately, most US adults do not consume the recommended amount of fiber per day. The Dietary Guidelines for Americans advise consuming about 14 grams of fiber per 1,000 calories. However, most adults benefit from eating much more than that regardless of the total number of calories they are consuming. *The Core Three Healthy Eating Plan recommends aiming for at least 25 grams of fiber per day.* Enjoying a variety of fiber is also important, as each type plays a different role in the body. The two most prominent types of fiber are soluble and insoluble.

### Soluble Fiber

Soluble fiber dissolves in water, forming a gel-like substance. Think of soluble fiber like a towel that soaks up cholesterol and fat, cleaning up the GI tract. Soluble fibers are often fermentable fibers that feed your gut healthy bacteria, strengthening your gut microbiome and increasing your metabolism. The best sources of soluble fiber include:

- Beans
- Lentils
- Oats
- Avocados
- Psyllium powder
- Partially hydrolyzed guar gum

### Insoluble Fiber

Insoluble fiber is not dissolvable and therefore acts more like a power wash, cleaning out your digestive tract, bulking up your stool, and pushing everything right along (bye-bye, constipation). For that reason, a high-insoluble-fiber diet can be protective against colon cancer as well.

The best sources of insoluble fiber are:

- Wheat bran
- Skins of fruits and veggies
- Beans
- Nuts
- Seeds

While fiber is a carbohydrate, it is also found in certain fats like nuts, seeds, non-starchy veggies, and certain types of plant protein foods. You will notice fiber content next to applicable foods in Chapters 5 and 6. This will help you easily keep track so you can reach your fiber needs for the day. The meal plans in Chapter 12 are also designed to incorporate higher-fiber foods into your diet.

### Resistant Starches

Resistant starches are a carbohydrate that, like fiber, resists digestion. Studies show that these slow-digesting starches act as prebiotics that feed the healthy bacteria in your gut, and foods higher in resistant starch keep blood sugar and insulin levels stable. A 2016 article published in the peer-reviewed journal *Scientific Reports* titled "Impact of Dietary Resistant Starch Type 4 on Human Gut Microbiota and Immunometabolic Functions" shows that resistant starches improved bacteria balance in the gut, which ultimately improved metabolism. Resistant starches are commonly found in potatoes, whole grains, and a variety of beans, as well as certain fruits like green bananas.

While heating can destroy resistant starch in potatoes and grains like oats and rice, once these foods are cooled, a new type of resistant starch is formed. This new type of starch is more resilient against heat; therefore, reheating the food after it has cooled does not destroy the starch again. To take advantage of this new type of starch, you can consider when and how you eat foods that contain it. For example, if you enjoy hot oatmeal in the morning, you can simply cook the oats the night before, store them in the fridge, and then warm them up again in the morning. Alternatively, you can prepare the Overnight Gut-Feeding Oats recipe in Chapter 13 and enjoy the oats cold. Since they are not heated, the original form of resistant starch is left intact.

### The Facts on Fruit

Fruit often gets a bad reputation because it contains simple carbs, or sugar. But it can actually be slow-digesting due to its higher fiber, antioxidant, and resistant starch content. Within the minimum three daily servings of carbohydrates on the Core Three Plan, it is important to include at least one serving of fruit for a well-rounded, all-inclusive diet.

Fruit can make for a convenient snack that helps satisfy a mild sweet tooth. Although fruit does contain sugar, predominantly in the form of fructose, it is a natural sugar that is digested differently than added, refined sugars are. Natural sugars also come packaged with a variety of health-promoting nutrients aside from fiber and resistant starch, such as immune-supporting vitamin C, potassium for healthy muscle function, and polyphenols that act as antioxidants fighting inflammation in your body.

Unlike other types of sugar found in carbohydrates, fructose does not immediately rush into your bloodstream. It is first shunted to your liver, where it is partially converted into glucose. It may then enter your bloodstream, where it can be used as energy or transported via insulin to your glycogen stores. This circuitous route is why many fruits, especially higher-fiber fruits like berries, have minimal impact on blood sugar levels.

Bananas, watermelon, mango, and pineapple also contain fructose but are slightly higher in sucrose and lower in fiber, which means they may have a more immediate impact on blood sugars. Regardless, the fact remains that you're still obtaining an array of nutrients from fresh fruit, which means it's a vital food group for balanced eating. As long as your total daily carbohydrates stay within the recommended guidelines, there is no need to avoid fruit or be afraid to enjoy it regularly.

## What Makes a Carb Faster-Digesting?

The more refined, processed, or sugary a carb is, the faster and easier it is to digest. Carbs with higher amounts of added sugars, like sodas, candy, syrups, and sweetened cereals, break down into glucose and enter your bloodstream more rapidly than other carbs. This leads to a spike in blood sugar and energy levels that plummet quickly after. Your body may then crave more sugar to restore energy levels. Eating sweet-tasting foods can also stimulate the pleasure center of your brain, which can explain why sugar cravings are so common.

The rate of digestion can be entirely dependent on the individual, but most will see a quicker spike in blood sugar, and thus insulin levels, after eating these types of carbs versus slower-digesting versions. It also depends on what other foods or nutrients are eaten at the same time. If you're eating full-fat ice cream, the fat can help slow down the rate at which you digest the sugar. Either way, you do not need to avoid all added sugar and processed carbs. While you can survive without these foods, it can be difficult to sustain this type of eating pattern in our world. The more you tell yourself that a food is off-limits, the more you may feel out of control around this food when it becomes available. You may find it helps to allow yourself a small piece of chocolate every once in a while to avoid getting carried away and eating an entire tray of cookies at the next holiday dinner.

Aside from added sugars, overly processed foods like refined white flours, white rice, added sugars or sweeteners, and syrups are basically predigested for you. For that reason, they spike blood sugars and insulin levels much faster, which can contribute to weight gain and intense sugar and carb cravings. The Core Three Plan promotes stable blood sugars and insulin, which will support your journey to finding your happy, healthy weight and feeling more energized.

## Why Some Dairy Can Be Considered a Carb

You will also notice that "milk and milk substitutes" fall under the carbohydrate category on the Core Three Healthy Eating Plan. This does not mean *all* dairy products are considered carbohydrates—just certain types of dairy, like milk and non-Greek-style yogurt. Milk specifically contains more natural sugar, in the form of lactose (another simple carb), than cheese. If you are lactose intolerant or lactose-sensitive, you might notice you cannot

### Sugar Addiction Confliction

Sugar addictions are a common discussion among the healthcare community. The risk factors for any addiction include genetics, age, environment, personality type, medical history, and mental health issues. The American Psychiatric Association defines addiction as a complex brain disease that is manifested by compulsive substance use despite harmful consequence. That definition alone, when applied to sugar, would lead you to believe that EATING SUGAR = HARMFUL CONSEQUENCE. The reality is that our bodies are designed to prefer sugar. Eating something sweet can activate the feel-good neurotransmitters in your brain, aka dopamine. That is because if your blood sugar gets low enough, it can lead to seizures, loss of consciousness, and even death. Thus, your body understands that sugar keeps you alive. Of course, you can get sugar from various foods, not just ice cream, chocolate, or candy. However, if you have been depriving yourself of food or trying to avoid carbs and sugar, your body might be trying to compensate. There is a clear distinction between bingeing on a pint of ice cream because you have been depriving your body of this comfort food for weeks and an unconditional sugar addiction. If your overwhelming sweet tooth is due to food deprivation, reintroducing small amounts is the best approach to thwart a compulsive sugar-seeking addiction. Otherwise, if you believe it is truly an addiction and not a response to restriction, practicing sugar avoidance may be the answer. But it is important to identify the root cause before acting.

tolerate milk in your cereal but can easily digest a cheese stick in the afternoon.

A 100-calorie serving of milk has an average of 12–15 grams of carbohydrates compared with just 1 gram of carbohydrate in a 100-calorie serving of cheese. Therefore, we put milk in the carbohydrate section and we consider cheese a protein—unless it is whole-milk cheese, in which case it becomes a fat.

In recent years, cheese and milk have come under fire as more consumers have heard about the supposed "dangers of dairy." Cancer, heart disease, and obesity are just a few of the many allegations lobbed against this cow-derived food group. Although responses will vary from person to person, most individuals need not be afraid of eating dairy. Dairy-based foods offer protein, calcium, vitamin D, and iodine, and yogurt and kefir are the richest sources of gut-friendly probiotics. Otherwise, there are only a few dairy-free options for obtaining these precious bugs: Kombucha, kimchi, miso, and tempeh are among the short list of nondairy probiotic-rich foods.

While you can obtain many of dairy's star nutrients in other foods like veggies, seafood, and plant milks, omitting any major food groups is not advised so you can build a healthier relationship with food. If you enjoy sprinkling Parmesan cheese on your roasted broccoli or like to have a yogurt with fresh berries as a quick breakfast, there is no need to stop. That said, if you notice immediate reactions that include digestive discomfort or skin issues after consuming milk, yogurt, or cheese, reducing your intake of cow's-milk dairy or replacing it with plant-based almond or coconut versions is perfectly fine. Ultimately, unless you are strictly plant-based or you have a known reaction to dairy or a special condition (which we will discuss later), do not shun dairy products.

## High-Fiber Carbohydrates Food Lists

The following charts list the Core Three portion sizes for various types of carbs, along with how many grams of fiber each contains. Use it to keep track of how much fiber you are eating every day—remember, the goal is at least 25 grams per day. You do not have to track this number religiously, but becoming familiar with fiber content can help you make healthier choices. You will notice that some foods contain a significant amount of fiber in just one serving. While they can easily help you reach your target for the day, you do want to be cautious about how much you consume in one meal or snack. To avoid stomach upset or irritability, I suggest not eating more than 15 grams of fiber in one shot. Instead, break it up into smaller portions, and always make sure to drink plenty of water when eating a higher-fiber food. The water will assist in pushing the fiber through your digestive tract and decrease any bloating or discomfort.

In the list that follows, you will also notice some carb choices that are lower in fiber, or under 5 grams per serving. It is important for food freedom that you have variety in your diet and do not feel limited to just high-fiber carbs. As long as you reach your fiber goals for the day, you can enjoy whatever options you prefer. There are also some foods not included in the list, like quick-digesting carbs. Since nothing is excluded on this plan, there is room for these types of foods through flexible carb options and discretionary meals, which will be explained later.

You will not see veggies like broccoli, spinach, carrots, beets, and celery in the list because they are non-starchy vegetables. (Those tables are shown in Chapter 7.) Whether your goal is to lose weight or not, I encourage you to enjoy them more liberally. As explained in Chapter 3, I recommend that you consume a MINIMUM of three servings of non-starchy veggies per day.

## Bread

| FOOD | FIBER | PORTION |
|---|---|---|
| Bagel, whole-grain | 2g | ⅓ bagel |
| Bread, whole-grain | 3g | 1 slice |
| Bread crumbs, whole-grain | 2g | ¼ cup |
| English muffin, light or 100-calorie | 5g | 1 whole |
| English muffin, regular | 1g | ½ muffin |
| Food for Life Sprouted Gluten-Free Bread (Almond, Flax) | 3–4g | 1 slice |
| Food for Life Sprouted Grain Bread (Flax) | 6g | 2 slices |
| Naan or roti, whole-wheat | 2g | 1 oz. |
| Pita, 6-inch whole-grain | 2g | ½ pita |
| Taco shell | 0g | 2 shells |
| Three Bakers Gluten-Free Golden Flax Bread | 4g | 1 slice |
| Tortilla, 7.5-inch whole-wheat | 4g | 1 tortilla |
| Trader Joe's Sprouted 7-Grain Bread | 4g | 2 slices |
| Udi's Gluten-Free Millet-Chia Bread | 5g | 2 slices |

## Cereals

| FOOD | FIBER | PORTION |
|---|---|---|
| Bran cereal* (Brands: Fiber One, Kashi GO, All-Bran) | 10–20g | 1 cup |
| Cereal bars* (Brands: Fiber One, Kashi) | 5–10g | 1 bar |
| Puffed wheat cereal | 3g | 1½ cups |
| Shredded wheat, plain | 3g | ½ cup (1 oz.) |
| Unsweetened, ready-to-eat cereal (Brands: Cheerios, Special K, Wheat Chex) | 0–2g | ¾ cup |

*Ideally look for cereal and cereal bars with less than 8g of sugar and greater than 5g of fiber per 15g of carbohydrates.

## Grains

| FOOD | FIBER | PORTION |
|------|-------|---------|
| Ancient Harvest quinoa pasta, cooked | 2g | ½ cup |
| Banza chickpea pasta, cooked (grain substitute) | 4g | ⅔ cup |
| Barilla gluten-free pasta, cooked | 1g | ½ cup |
| Barley, cooked | 5g | ½ cup |
| Farro, cooked | 3g | ½ cup |
| Fiber Gourmet pasta, cooked | 25g | 1 cup |
| Kasha, cooked | 2g | ½ cup |
| Millet, cooked | 2g | ½ cup |
| Oats, regular or quick, dry | 3g | 6 Tbsp. |
| Oats, steel-cut, dry | 3g | 3 Tbsp. |
| Quinoa, cooked (any color) | 3g | ½ cup |
| Rice, brown, cooked | 2g | ½ cup |
| Rice, red, cooked | 1g | ½ cup |
| Teff, cooked | 2g | ½ cup |
| Tolerant organic red lentil pasta, cooked (grain substitute) | 3g | ½ cup |
| Wheat germ, dry | 4g | 3 Tbsp. |
| Whole-wheat pasta, cooked | 2g | ½ cup |

## Crackers and Snacks

| FOOD | FIBER | PORTION |
| --- | --- | --- |
| Matzo, egg | 1g | 1 sheet |
| Matzo, light whole-wheat bran | 9g | 1½ sheets |
| Popcorn, air-popped, no butter or oil added | 1g | 4 cups |
| Rice cakes, 60-calorie | 3g | 2 cakes |
| Ryvita Multigrain Crackers | 6g | 3 crackers |
| Wasa Crackers, Original or Rye | 8g | 3 crackers |
| Wasa, Light Rye | 6g | 4 crackers |

## Starchy Veggies

All the servings are for cooked vegetables—non-starchy vegetables are unlimited and will be discussed later.

| FOOD | FIBER | PORTION |
| --- | --- | --- |
| Cassava | 0g | ⅓ cup |
| Corn | 5g | ⅔ cup |
| Green peas | 7g | 1 cup |
| Plantains | 2.5g | ½ cup |
| Potato, white | 2g | 1 small baked/boiled |
| Pumpkin puree, canned, no sugar added | 6g | 1 cup |
| Squash, acorn | 9g | ½ cup |
| Squash, butternut | 3g | 1 cup |
| Sweet potato or yam | 4g | 1 medium |
| Tomato sauce, store-bought, jarred | 2–4g | 1 cup |

## Legumes (based on cooked portions)

| FOOD | FIBER | PORTION |
| --- | --- | --- |
| Black beans | 6g | ⅔ cup |
| Garbanzo beans (chickpeas) | 6g | ⅔ cup |
| Kidney beans | 9g | ⅔ cup |
| Lentils, cooked (any color) | 11g | ⅔ cup |
| Lima beans | 7g | ⅔ cup |
| Peas, black-eyed or split | 5g | ⅔ cup |
| Pinto beans | 13g | ⅔ cup |
| Refried beans | 6g | ⅔ cup |
| Soybeans (edamame) | 6g | ⅔ cup |
| White beans | 8g | ⅔ cup |

## Fruits

Stick with mostly fresh fruit, rather than dried or juiced, as it can be more filling, voluminous, and fiber-rich.

| FOOD | FIBER | PORTION |
| --- | --- | --- |
| Apple | 4g | 1 medium |
| Apples, dried | 3g | 5 rings |
| Applesauce, unsweetened | 4g | ⅔ cup |
| Apricots, fresh | 3g | 5 apricots |
| Banana | 3g | 1 small |
| Blackberries | 11g | 1¾ cups |
| Blueberries | 4g | 1¼ cups fresh, 1 cup frozen |
| Cantaloupe | 2g | 1½ cups |
| Cherries, fresh | 3g | 1¼ cups |

| FOOD | FIBER | PORTION |
|------|-------|---------|
| Dates, dried | 2g | 4 small |
| Dried fruits (berries, cherries, raisins) | 2g | 1 oz. |
| Figs, fresh | 4g | 2 medium |
| Grapefruit, fresh | 4g | 1 whole |
| Grapes | 1g | ⅔ cup |
| Guava | 6g | 2½ small |
| Honeydew melon | 2g | 1½ cups |
| Kiwi | 4g | 2 medium |
| Mango | 3g | 1 cup fresh, ⅔ cup frozen |
| Nectarine | 1g | 2 small |
| Orange | 3g | 1 medium |
| Papaya | 5g | 1 small |
| Peaches | 4g | 2 small |
| Pear | 6–8g | 1 medium |
| Pineapple | 1g | ⅔ cup fresh, ½ cup frozen |
| Plums, fresh | 3g | 3 small |
| Pomegranate seeds | 4g | ⅔ cup |
| Raspberries | 12g | 1½ cups fresh, ⅔ cup frozen |
| Strawberries | 6g | 2 cups fresh, 1¼ cups frozen |
| Tangerine | 2g | 2 small |
| Watermelon | 1g | 1 cup |

## Milk and Milk Substitutes

| FOOD | FIBER | PORTION |
| --- | --- | --- |
| Almond milk, unsweetened | 1g/cup | Free |
| Coconut milk, unsweetened | 1g/cup | Free |
| Cow's milk, 0–4% | 0g | 1 cup |
| Hemp milk, unsweetened | 1g/cup | Free |
| Oat milk, plain | 2g | 1 cup |
| Soy milk, unsweetened | 1g | 1 cup |
| Yogurt, almond or coconut milk, unsweetened | 2g | ¾ cup |
| Yogurt, plain (non-Greek), unsweetened* | 0g | 1 cup |
| Yogurt, oat milk, unsweetened | 2g | 1 cup |
| Yogurt, soy milk, unsweetened | 1g | 1 cup |

* Sweeten your yogurts naturally with fresh fruit, cinnamon, vanilla extract, and cocoa powder.

Now that you understand the importance of consuming high-fiber carbohydrates and how they fit into the Core Three, you can work on developing a healthier relationship with the foods you enjoy eating. An integral step in this process is discovering what is behind your carb cravings and why you may eat more than you need. Although eating excessive amounts of carbs (or anything for that matter) can lead to weight gain over time, this is more likely to occur if you're eating an imbalanced diet that is devoid of fiber and nutrients. Overly restricting and avoiding carbs is not the solution. Fortunately, you now have this list to help guide your food choices while you learn how to eat for your body. Remember, the higher the fiber, the longer you remain full. Core Three carbs truly provide the finest fuel our bodies demand. In the next chapter, we will discuss the second pillar of the Core Three: lean proteins.

# Lean Proteins

A higher-protein diet is usually the difference between losing weight and maintaining weight. Yet most people don't eat enough of this core macronutrient. According to the National Health and Nutrition Examination Survey, Americans consume only 16 percent of their total calories from protein. That means 84 percent of calories are carbs and fats, leading to an imbalance of energy that can pack on pounds. Why? Protein is not prioritized. Eating more protein-rich foods is crucial for health and to find your healthiest, happiest weight.

Protein fills you up, feeds lean muscle to spark fat-burning, and offers essential energizing nutrients. It is the gateway to growth and repair, providing amino acids (which are the building blocks in your body). These amino acids build up your muscles and connective tissues and help stabilize blood sugars and boost neurotransmitters that regulate mood and appetite.

This chapter will provide an overview of lean proteins, what they are, and why they are an essential macronutrient in the Core Three Healthy Eating Plan. You will learn about various sources of lean protein and why a variety of both plant and animal protein foods is ideal. We will also discuss how much protein to eat in a day. If you're vegetarian or vegan, I will explain how to adjust the plan to fit your needs. I will also touch upon processed protein foods and protein supplements, including bars and collagen powders. Finally, you will receive a detailed list of Core Three lean proteins to focus on for optimal health and well-being.

## What Are Lean Proteins?

Typically "lean" proteins refers to fat content, and indeed, most Core Three lean proteins are lower in inflammatory fat. But the Core Three Healthy Eating Plan goes beyond that and also uses this term to describe more nutritious, energizing, fulfilling, and health-promoting proteins. Including a variety of Core Three protein foods supports freedom of choice.

The US Department of Agriculture specifically defines "lean proteins" as "having less than 10 grams of total fat, 4.5 grams or less of saturated fat, and less than 95 milligrams of cholesterol" in a 3.5-ounce portion. For example, a lean protein option is chicken breast, which has less than 1 gram of saturated fat per 4-ounce serving, compared with chicken legs, which have 12 grams of saturated fat for the same quantity. Fat is not "bad," but saturated fats are more pro-inflammatory and artery-clogging. (The next chapter will provide an overview of anti-inflammatory versus pro-inflammatory fats.)

Fattier cuts of animal proteins, especially red meat, can raise LDL cholesterol levels and increase the risk of heart disease—the leading cause of death in the US, above cancer. (The next chapter will provide more information on cholesterol as well. Refined carbohydrates, including added sugars, are also a causal factor of heart disease. Hence, the healthiest diet embraces a balance of higher-fiber, less-processed carbs; lean proteins; and anti-inflammatory fats.)

### Higher-Fat Proteins and Omega-3s

You will notice that several higher-fat proteins are recommended in the Core Three Healthy Eating Plan, including fatty cold-water-sourced fish like salmon and tuna, as well as wild or grass-fed meat. These types of proteins offer a valuable source of omega-3 fatty acids, which we will discuss in the next chapter. *Consuming fatty fish only three times a week provides you with all the omega-3s you need for an entire week.* You will find recipes in Chapters 13–15 to help you incorporate more fatty fish into your diet.

## Why Lean on Lean Proteins?

Foods like chicken breast, eggs, Greek yogurt, tofu, and beans are more nutritious choices than other foods—such as quick-digesting carbohydrates—that may contribute to blood sugar crashes and body fat storage. Protein-rich foods are more like slow-digesting carbs, as they are also harder to break down. They offer the best source of immune-boosting zinc, energizing B vitamins, and blood-pumping iron.

A higher-protein diet also:

- **Promotes fullness:** According to a 2004 review published in the *Journal of the American College of Nutrition*, "there is convincing evidence that a higher protein intake increases thermogenesis and satiety compared to diets of lower protein content." Thermogenesis is the process by which your body burns fuel, and potentially body fat, to produce heat. It is a necessary part of body maintenance and energy balance. Not only can protein burn more energy during digestion than other types of macronutrients, but protein-rich foods can influence specific hormones, such as ghrelin and PYY, that regulate hunger and appetite. Ultimately, protein may decrease hunger-inducing hormones and increase hormones that lead to feelings of fullness.

- **Mitigates muscle loss:** A 2008 review printed in the *Journal of the American Dietetic Association* finds "inadequate protein intake during caloric restriction may be associated with adverse body-composition changes." Losing some muscle while losing weight may be unavoidable, but adequate protein consumption can reduce or prevent this process and encourage more fat-burning instead. The more muscle you have, the more efficient your metabolism runs, because muscle is a metabolically active tissue that guzzles more fuel (or calories) during activity and rest.
- **Balances blood sugars:** Protein directly supports, and is often necessary for, muscle growth. Lean muscle directly enhances insulin function. Insulin, in turn, regulates blood sugar levels. Therefore, adequate protein intake is important for body composition, or increased muscle mass, and thus blood sugar regulation.
- **Provides energy:** Although carbohydrates are still our premier source of fuel, protein can also be converted into energy. Protein foods also contribute the best source of nutrients that directly support healthy energy levels: iron, B vitamins, vitamin D, iodine, zinc, and amino acids.

## What Makes a Protein Essential?

Protein contains all nine essential amino acids (or organic compounds), which we cannot manufacture on our own:

- **Histidine:** assists with production of histamine, an important neurotransmitter that regulates immune response, digestion, and sleep
- **Isoleucine:** a component in muscle growth and energy regulation
- **Leucine:** assists with muscle repair and blood sugar balance
- **Lysine:** important for hormone, energy, and collagen production
- **Methionine:** a key player in metabolism and detoxification, also necessary

for absorption of zinc and selenium, vital nutrients for thyroid function and fighting oxidative stress

- **Phenylalanine:** a precursor for feel-good neurotransmitters in our brains like dopamine, epinephrine, and norepinephrine
- **Threonine:** an integral part of structural proteins like collagen and elastin that support all connective tissues in our bodies; also influences fat metabolism and immune function
- **Tryptophan:** precursor of serotonin that regulates appetite, sleep, and mood
- **Valine:** stimulates muscle growth and contributes to energy production

A variety of protein-rich foods will ensure adequate absorption of each of these amino acids to help keep you healthy and strong.

## Animal Protein and Plant Protein

Proteins are classified into two categories: animal and plant. Both are included in the Core Three Plan. Animal proteins include poultry, fish, beef, pork, dairy, eggs, and wild game. Protein-rich plant foods include tofu, beans, lentils, and vegan protein powders made from peas, soy, or seeds.

## The Benefits of Blending Both Proteins

Of course, you can choose not to eat any animal products for moral or religious reasons. However, from a health perspective, it is beneficial to eat a blend or balance of animal *and* plant proteins. Animal proteins offer more absorbable forms of amino acids, blood-pumping iron, immune-supporting zinc and vitamin D, energizing B vitamins, and bone-building calcium. They are inherently complete, offering all nine essential amino acids that your body can't manufacture on its own. Plant proteins also supply vital nutrients like fiber, antioxidants, magnesium, and iron, but very few are considered complete proteins. Therefore, you need to include more plant proteins—like whole grains, beans, lentils, nuts, and seeds—to eat a higher-protein diet.

Keep in mind that calories from animal-based food sources like grilled chicken or fish are almost entirely protein. While calories from plant-food sources like beans, grains, nuts, and seeds do provide protein, they are predominantly carbohydrates and fats. Thus, balancing macros is harder when you're strictly plant-based. For example, a 4-ounce serving of boneless chicken breast supplies about 20 grams of complete protein and around 125 calories. To obtain the same amount of protein from peanut butter, you would need to eat 6 tablespoons, which also provides 50 grams of fat and

### Wild about Wild Proteins

Farmed and conventionally raised animals live a more confined life and are fed a grain-based diet. This leads to lower amounts of anti-inflammatory omega-3 fatty acids and higher amounts of pro-inflammatory omega-6 fatty acids, which can increase the risk of certain diseases such as diabetes and heart disease. Wild and grass-fed animals eat a grass-based diet and live a more active lifestyle, which increases the favorable anti-inflammatory omega-3 fatty acids. This *wilder* lifestyle can also increase other nutrients, such as disease-fighting antioxidants and vitamin D. Like grass-fed beef, wild seafood offers more anti-inflammatory fats. Studies also show wild salmon has fewer contaminants, such as PCBs, than farmed fish that live in enclosed, controlled environments.

Why not always choose wild? Some find that the taste and consistency are not as enjoyable. Wild fish and beef can also be pricier and potentially harder to find. Ultimately, if you can overcome these hurdles, choose wild over farmed or grain-fed, but the end goal is to make sure you're eating sufficient protein in balance with other Core Three macros.

580 calories—more than four times the amount in chicken.

Incorporating both types of protein can make it easier to balance your macronutrients—an integral step in the Core Three. Regardless, a successful diet must accommodate your specific needs, preferences, and lifestyle.

### Personalizing the Core Three for Plant Eaters

Plant-based, animal-free diets are a frontline solution to environmental sustainability and the health of our planet. However, relying only on plant foods makes it tricky to limit your carb and fat intake. That said, if you are a vegan or vegetarian, you can still follow this plan and achieve your goals. Veganism does require a little extra

planning, but it can be healthy. There is a Core Three vegan meal plan in Chapter 12 that provides insight on how to balance your plant-based diet. Vegans should also receive routine blood checkups to ensure sufficient levels of iron and vitamin D. A multivitamin can help fill in nutritional gaps, as well as an algae oil supplement for essential, anti-inflammatory omega 3 fatty acids.

### Dairy Protein

Most dairy products provide protein in two forms: whey and casein. Casein is a slower-digesting protein that takes time for full absorption. Whey is a faster-digesting protein that can increase insulin when consumed in larger quantities, similar to certain carbs. Both are considered complete proteins and offer all nine essential amino acids.

Milk and regular yogurt are considered carbs because of their elevated natural sugar content in the form of lactose. On the other hand, Greek yogurt and light, or reduced-fat, cheese contain more protein, in the form of whey and casein, than carbs. These dairy foods are also a leading source of calcium, vitamin D, and iodine, and yogurt is the best source of gut-friendly probiotics.

If you don't eat dairy and prefer almond milk– or coconut milk–based yogurts, these do not supply the same amount of protein. Along with full-fat cheese, plant-based yogurts are considered fats and will be listed in the next chapter. Full-fat cheese is also not on the list of protein foods because it has more calories from fat than protein. No matter what, all types of dairy and plant-based dairy alternatives have a place in this plan. You can pick and choose which options best suit your preferences.

## The Collagen Craze

What exactly is collagen? It is a type of protein found naturally in our connective tissues, such as tendons, muscles, and skin, that acts like a glue, holding our bodies together. Around age 20–30, we start to

### Animal Protein and the Environment

When meat is cultivated, particularly from cows, it can burn through a disproportionate amount of water compared with what's used to grow fruits and veggies. Animal products also exhaust natural resources and increase greenhouse gases that exacerbate climate change. Even seafood farming and fishing practices have been linked to harming the planet's welfare. The Dietary Guidelines for Americans now advise consumers to eat more plant-based foods and cut down on meat and animal proteins. In 2007, the Academy of Nutrition and Dietetics encouraged "environmentally responsible practices that conserve natural resources, minimize the quantity of waste generated, and support the ecological sustainability of the food system." We rely on our planet for nutritious food, so considering environmental sustainability is ultimately good for our health as well.

naturally lose collagen through aging— roughly 1 percent per year. The result is thinner skin that shows wrinkles and fine lines and feels dehydrated.

Collagen supplements have become very popular, reaching an all-time high of $46.6 million in sales in 2018, increasing nearly 34 percent from 2017. Why all the hype? Studies show that collagen may help fight the effects of aging; improve skin elasticity, hair, and nails; and diminish joint pain or inflammation. One of the biggest assertions is gut health improvement, including a strengthening of the lining in your digestive tract.

Collagen is composed of nineteen amino acids—but only eight of the nine essential amino acids—that assist in rebuilding and repair (much like any other protein you eat). Theoretically, dietary collagen can directly strengthen the collagen in your body, but study results are mixed and research is still inconclusive. We know that after ingestion collagen breaks down into individual amino acids that travel wherever they're needed, healing skin, growing hair, producing hormone, or repairing muscles. Whether you're getting these amino acids directly from a collagen supplement or from another protein source like fish, cheese, eggs, or quinoa, eating sufficient protein can help with collagen production in your body.

Dietary collagen is commonly found in animal muscle (as opposed to organ meats), as well as eggs, fish, bone broth, and spirulina. Is it still worth taking a collagen supplement, especially if you're already eating collagen-rich foods? It can be, and it certainly won't hurt. More research is required to determine whether collagen is a useful additive. However, if you already have sufficient protein in your diet, which of course you will with the Core Three Healthy Eating Plan, it is not a *necessary* addition to your routine.

## Animal-Based Lean Proteins

When looking at protein food labels, one serving equals about 100–150 calories and an average of 20 grams of protein. The measurements are based on dry weight of raw, uncooked meat/fish if you're weighing on a food scale. Or you can figure it out by the package. There are 16 ounces in 1 pound, so if you're buying 1 pound of fish, you can figure there are about five 3-ounce portions.

| FOOD | PORTION |
| --- | --- |
| Beef, grass-fed or conventional, ground (90 percent lean or higher; select or choice grades) (Trimmed of fat: roast—chuck, round, rump, sirloin.) | 3 oz. |
| Beef jerky (Limit beef jerky if you have a history of hypertension, because it's a high-sodium food.) | 1½ oz. |
| Cheese, cottage or ricotta, light, part-skim, reduced-fat, or fat-free | 1 cup |
| Cheese, light, part-skim, or fat-free (Full-fat cheese is not listed here, as it's considered a fat. Although fat-free is listed, it is typically less satisfying than higher-fat versions.) | 3 oz. |
| Deli meat (turkey, ham, roast beef, chicken) (These are considered processed meats that are higher in sodium and nitrates.) | 4 oz. |
| Eggs (If you have a history of cardiovascular disease, high cholesterol, or high triglycerides, stick with 3–5 whole eggs per week. You can also combine 1 whole egg + 4 egg whites to make it 1 protein serving without the excess saturated fat.) | 2 whole eggs + 2 egg whites |
| Egg substitutes | ½ cup |
| Egg whites | 1 cup or 7 egg whites |
| Fish (cod, flounder, halibut, orange roughy, sole, tilapia) | 4 oz. |

| FOOD | PORTION |
| --- | --- |
| Fish, oily (anchovies, herring, trout, salmon, sardines, tuna—fresh, smoked, cured, or canned) (Aim for three servings per week to get the recommended amount of anti-inflammatory omega-3 fatty acids. Choose wild when possible.) | 3 oz. |
| Game, grass-fed or conventional (buffalo, ostrich, rabbit, venison) | 3 oz. |
| Goat | 4 oz. |
| Lean ground turkey or chicken (at least 90 percent lean) | 4 oz. |
| Oysters, fresh or frozen | 18 oysters |
| Pork (ham, rib, or loin chop/roast, tenderloin) | 4 oz. |
| Poultry, breast, boneless, skinless (white meat chicken breast, Cornish hen, turkey breast) | 4 oz. |
| Shellfish (clams, crab, lobster, scallops, shrimp) | 5 oz. |
| Steak, grass-fed or conventional, cubed (flank, porterhouse, T-bone, tenderloin) | 3 oz. |
| Veal, cutlet (no breading), loin chop, or roast | 3 oz. |
| Yogurt, Greek-style, unsweetened (full-fat, reduced-fat, 2%, or low-fat) | 6 oz. |

## Proteins Not on This List

If you don't see a particular protein food listed, that does not mean it is off-limits. Fattier cuts of meat that are not included—like chicken wings, pork chops, or rib-eye steak—are higher in pro-inflammatory fat. Breakfast meats like sausage and bacon, even when in chicken or turkey form, are considerably higher in fat, sodium, and nitrates. They can still be enjoyed in your weekly discretionary meals, which will be discussed in a future chapter.

### Higher-Fat Proteins

It is fine to enjoy higher-fat proteins two to three times per week in 3-ounce portions. If you have a history of high cholesterol, high triglycerides, heart disease, or diabetes, however, it is best to limit them to one time per week. Frequent consumption of red meat, particularly beef, pork, and lamb, can lead to more health risks, such as cancer.

Any land animal meat that has *5 grams of fat or more per 1 ounce raw* can be counted as follows: *1 fat and 1 protein per 3 ounces*. This includes dark meat chicken and turkey, 85 percent lean beef, and fattier cuts of steak and pork. Although it can be counted in the total fat for the day, it is prudent to limit saturated fat. This will be discussed more in the next chapter.

## Processed Meats

Specific deli meats are included in the list, although they are higher in nitrates and sodium. (Other processed protein foods—bacon, sausage, and hot dogs—are not included because they're higher-fat proteins.) Either way, all processed meats involve a degree of curing, smoking, or salting or contain added preservatives. They can all be hazardous to your health when eaten in larger quantities. The American Institute of Cancer Research reports that "every 50 grams (about one hot dog or two slices of ham) eaten daily raises the risk of colorectal cancer by 16 percent."

Overconsuming processed meats has also been linked to other forms of cancer and heart disease. Even if the package says "reduced-fat," "uncured," or "no antibiotics," the product is not much healthier. Uncured hot dogs are still high in sodium and saturated fat, and they may still contain carcinogenic nitrates. For that reason, it is safest to limit consumption of processed meats to a maximum of one to two times per month.

## Plant-Based Proteins

Aim for at least *two to three strictly plant-based meals per week*, whether you're a vegan or not.

| FOOD | PORTION | FIBER | SERVINGS |
|------|---------|-------|----------|
| Beans (black, garbanzo, kidney, lima, pinto, white), cooked or canned | 1½ cups | 12–21g | 1 protein + 2 carbs |
| Beans (navy, pinto, white, soybeans), cooked or canned | 1½ cups | 12–21g | 1 protein + 2 carbs |
| "Beef" or "sausage" crumbles, meatless | ⅔ cup | 5g | 1 protein |
| Beyond Meat Burger (Although it is plant-based, this is considered an ultra-processed product. It is higher in sodium and saturated fat. Best to limit food products like these to once a week.) | 4 oz. | 2g | 1 protein + 2 fats |
| Beyond Meat Crumbles (Although it is plant-based, this is considered an ultra-processed product. It is higher in sodium and saturated fat. Best to limit food products like these to once a week.) | ⅔ cup | 2g | 1 protein + ½ fat |
| Lentils, cooked or canned | 1½ cups | 24g | 1 protein + 2 carbs |
| Meatless Meatballs, Trader Joe's* | 7 meatballs | 5g | 1 protein + ½ fat |
| Nutritional yeast, Red Star brand | ¼ cup | 10g | 1 protein |
| Tempeh, plain/unflavored | 3 oz. | 3g | 1 protein + 1 fat |
| Tofu, firm or silken | ⅔ cup, uncooked | 1g | 1 protein + ½ fat |
| Veggie burger, BOCA Original* | 2 patties | 5g | 1½ proteins |

| FOOD | PORTION | FIBER | SERVINGS |
|------|---------|-------|----------|
| Veggie burger, Dr. Praeger's Perfect Burger* | 1 patty | 4g | 1 protein + 1 fat |
| Burger Patty, Impossible (Although it is plant-based, this is considered an ultra-processed product. It is higher in sodium and saturated fat. Best to limit food products like these to once a week.) | 4 oz. | 0g | 1 protein + 2 fats |

\* High in sodium.

## Protein Supplements

When it comes to nutrition, it is beneficial to get your nutrients from *food first.* Food is inherently balanced, offering a valuable and safe dose of everything you need. However, many people struggle to eat 25–35 percent of their total calories per day from protein. In those cases, supplements can help you hit your protein targets and fill in any nutritional gaps. They also make eating protein more convenient. For example, protein powders and bars are easily portable on busy days and while traveling. They can also help manage cravings and potentially satisfy a mild sweet tooth.

It's important you do not rely primarily on these supplements for protein. They are meant to *supplement* your diet, not replace it. Many proteins bars can cause gastrointestinal discomfort due to the added fiber and sweeteners. If you notice that is the case, you may want to avoid them and stick with whole-food protein sources. Either way, if you are eating protein bars every day or more than once a day, it is time to explore other options. If protein bars, especially sweeter-tasting versions, amplify your craving for additional sweets, limit your intake.

Protein powders can be mixed into smoothies or shakes and also be added to cooked or overnight oats. They help you meet your protein servings for the day to stay on plan. A portion is 20 grams of protein and around 100 calories. Scoop size will vary by brand, so look at the nutrition label and see how many scoops equal that amount (roughly 20 grams).

### Recommended Core Three Protein Powders
The following brands have reliable, safe, and quality ingredients. The Food and

Drug Administration (FDA) does not regulate supplements; however, companies such as ConsumerLab perform independent quality testing that is made available to the public. Many (but not all) of the products listed here have been verified by third-party companies to ensure the content of each product matches what is listed on the ingredients list and label. Third-party testing also ensures that there are no dangerous levels of any toxic heavy metals, which can be an issue with many protein powders.

### WHEY PROTEIN

- Brands: Naked Whey, Garden of Life, Designer Whey, Orgain, Power Crunch, Optimum Gold Standard 100% Whey, Vital Proteins

### VEGAN PROTEINS

- Brands: OWYN, Orgain, Garden of Life, Vega One, Nuzest

### READY-TO-DRINK SHAKES

- Vegan: OWYN, Vega Protein Nutrition Shake, Evolve Plant-Based Protein Shake
- Whey: ICONIC Protein Drink, Orgain Clean Protein Shake

## Recommended Protein Bars

Since many protein bars also contain other ingredients and are not strictly proteins, they will count as 1 protein and potentially 1 carb and/or 1 fat. See the Protein Bars table for reference.

## Protein Bars

| BRAND | FIBER | SERVINGS |
| --- | --- | --- |
| Atlas Bars | 11g | 1 protein + 1 fat (0 carb) |
| Garden of Life Fit Protein Bars | 13g | ½ protein + ½ carb + ½ fat |
| Garden of Life Performance Protein Bars | 10g | 1 protein + 1½ carbs + 1 fat |
| GNC Lean Bars | 8g | 1 protein + 1 carb |
| good! Snacks Bars | 11g | 1 protein + 1 carb + ½ fat |
| Kirkland Signature Protein Bars | 15g | 1 protein (0 carb) + ½ fat |
| No Cow Bars | 19g | 1 protein + ½ fat (0 carb) |
| ONE PLANT Protein Bars | 8g | ½ protein + ½ fat (0 carb) |
| Quest Bars | 15g | 1 protein + 1 fat (0 carb) |
| Raw Rev Glo Bars | 13g | ½ protein + 1 fat (0 carb) |

Lean proteins are an integral element in the success of the Core Three Healthy Eating Plan. If you're not a big protein eater, or you're a vegan and not used to eating large quantities of proteins, it could take additional planning to ensure you reach your daily goals. Remember that the more you add, the better you'll feel as your diet naturally becomes more well rounded. Along with strength training, a protein-rich diet will preserve lean body mass, ultimately driving metabolism and helping you feel your best. In the next chapter we'll take a closer look at fats, the final core macronutrient your body needs.

# CHAPTER 6

# Anti-Inflammatory Fats

Let's cut to the chase: Eating more fat will not make you "fatter." In fact, eating fats won't increase body fat stores any more than eating carbohydrates or proteins can—the real cause of weight gain is eating more than your body needs for fuel. Speaking of fuel, fat is also a fantastic source of energizing nutrients. Fats add flavor to meals, making them tastier; keep you feeling satiated; and help with fat-soluble vitamin absorption. Like fiber, fats also help slow down digestion and regulate blood sugars and insulin levels.

So, why are fats often limited and even avoided on weight loss diets? What would a salad be without a salad dressing, and how much more enjoyable is an apple or banana when it is dipped into a peanut butter spread? While it might seem easy to overdo it on fats like olive oil, avocado, and nut butters, this essential macronutrient amps up the satisfaction factor. Feeling satisfied with your food choices dampens pestering cravings and the urge to overeat. Incorporating more anti-inflammatory fats into your diet naturally keeps portions in check—no manipulation required. That is why they are a key macronutrient in the Core Three Healthy Eating Plan: They don't just fight inflammation; they facilitate finding your healthiest, happiest weight.

In this chapter, we will review the fundamentals of anti-inflammatory fats and why they are recommended on the Core Three. We will dive into the concept of inflammation and how fats contribute to this innate bodily response. I will break down why fats are important in general, especially for fighting inflammation and disease and promoting healthy weight management and energy. We will swim through the murky waters surrounding saturated fats and heart disease, as well as examine various types of fats and how some will fight inflammation more than others. We will uncover all you need to know about omega-3 fatty acids and why the ratio of omega-3 fatty acids to omega-6 fatty acids you eat can make a huge impact on your health and well-being, especially for fighting inflammation. We will briefly touch upon fats in your blood and how your diet can affect cholesterol levels and triglycerides. Finally, you will learn how much fat to consume and whether it's possible to overconsume fats, and you will receive a simplified and detailed list of Core Three fats to incorporate into your eating plan.

## What Are Fats?

As with carbs and proteins, not all fats are created equal. Some fats are more advantageous than others when it comes to health, energy, and weight management. The Core Three Plan groups fats by what they can do for your body—are they anti- or pro-inflammatory? There are predominantly four types of dietary fats: monounsaturated fatty acids (MUFAs), polyunsaturated fatty acids (PUFAs), saturated fats, and trans fats. Anti-inflammatory fats (generally, the MUFAs and PUFAs) fight inflammation in your body. They are more heart-protective and fiber-rich than other types of fats. Saturated and trans fats, on the other hand, are considered more pro-inflammatory.

The type of fat has nothing to do with total calories and grams. A tablespoon of olive oil has roughly the same calories and fat grams as a tablespoon of butter.

## What Is Inflammation?

Simply put, inflammation is your body's natural response to irritation or damage, like breathing in allergens or getting an insect bite. The point of this involuntary response is to initiate healing and recovery; however, it can be a double-edged sword. Inflammation starts as a helpful reaction, but when it persists, becomes widespread, and goes into overdrive, it can become

harmful. Signs of short-term inflammation include pain, redness, swelling, or heat at the affected site. Long-term, chronic inflammation, on the other hand, is systemic, can stay active for months and years, and leads to preventable diseases like diabetes, cardiovascular disease, and cancer. How do you know if you have persistent inflammation? Generally, you will have higher levels of C-reactive protein (CRP) detectable in your blood via a blood test.

Certain risk factors can make you more prone to inflammation and higher CRP levels, such as advanced age, higher body fat levels, excessive or insufficient exercise, smoking, stress, gut microbiota, and inadequate sleep—but the biggest risk factor is, of course, diet. When it comes to food, studies show that filling up on more refined carbohydrates and sugars, along with pro-inflammatory fats like saturated and trans fats, can contribute to persistent inflammation. A 2017 study published in the *Journal of Clinical Investigation*, titled "Hypothalamic Inflammation in Obesity and Metabolic Disease," reveals that "SFAs [saturated fatty acids], unlike unsaturated fatty acids, trigger the activation of inflammatory signaling" that contributes to a cascade of events such as insulin and leptin resistance. Insulin, we know from previous chapters, has a direct impact on body fat burning and appetite. Leptin is a hunger-satiating hormone that, when released, signals your brain to "put a fork in it because I have had enough to eat." A leptin resistance can make you feel like you're chasing your hunger all day long. In contrast, according to the same study, "unsaturated fatty acids, namely omega-3 fatty acids, restore leptin and insulin sensitivity." Ultimately, eating more anti-inflammatory foods can protect you from the hazards of chronic inflammatory markers that lead to appetite, weight, and health complications.

## Types of Fats

For the sake of fighting inflammation, strengthening insulin function, defending health, and promoting longevity, science still promotes consuming more MUFAs and PUFAs over saturated and trans fatty acids, with a special attention to omega-3s. Basically, prioritize the fats with the funky-sounding acronyms: MUFAs and omega-3-rich PUFAs! These are the anti-inflammatory fats. Let's learn more about each type.

### Monounsaturated Fatty Acids (MUFAs)

MUFAs are leaders in fighting inflamma-tion and for heart protection. They have a positive impact on cholesterol levels, energy, and blood sugar. Examples of MUFAs include olive oil, avocados, nuts, and seeds. Studies reveal that MUFA-rich foods can decrease heart attack–contrib-uting LDL cholesterol and increase heart health–promoting HDL cholesterol. One of the most well-regarded MUFAs

is extra-virgin olive oil, the celebrity of plant oils. This Mediterranean staple has the highest antioxidant activity (more on this activity later in this chapter), which directly lowers inflammation.

### Polyunsaturated Fatty Acids (PUFAs)

Most PUFAs are also considered anti-inflammatory. PUFAs include omega-3 and omega-6 fatty acids, which are both considered "essential" because our bodies cannot manufacture them. PUFAs are necessary for cell membrane structure, brain function, metabolism, reproductive health, and energy.

#### OMEGA-3S

You can find omega-3s in oily cold-water fish like anchovies, herring, mackerel, salmon, sardines, and tuna, as well as in algae and, in smaller amounts, in grass-fed cattle. Nuts and seeds like walnuts, pumpkin seeds, and chia seeds also contain omega-3s but in a slightly different form that is not as easily absorbed and beneficial.

#### OMEGA-6S

Omega-6s, on the other hand, are a more ubiquitous fat in the American diet. They are mostly consumed in the form of veg-etable oils (safflower, sunflower, peanut, canola, corn, soybean, sesame), vegetable oil spreads (mayo, margarine, butter sub-stitutes), certain nuts, and conventionally raised animal products. Fried foods are also a major source of omega-6 fatty acids. While most PUFAs are considered a "healthier fat," omega-6s' health effects on the body are conditional. Even though omega-6s are essential, consuming many more omega-6s than omega-3s can increase inflammation in the body, meaning these fats are no longer anti-inflammatory. Results from a 2018 Japanese study published in the *Journal of Internal Medicine*, based on 225 Japanese patients with type 2 diabetes, discovered that a diet high in omega-6 fatty acids may contribute to excess body fat accumulation and insulin resistance.

**BALANCING OMEGA-3S AND -6S**

The ideal ratio of omega-6 to omega-3 to fight disease is one to one, but statistics reveal that most adults in the US consume a ratio closer to twenty to one. A 2016 study published in the journal *Nutrients* found that this unbalanced ratio of omega-6 to omega-3 promotes inflammation, which contributes to conditions including atherosclerosis (a buildup of fat and/or cholesterol in the arteries), obesity, and diabetes. A 2002 review titled "The Importance of the Ratio of Omega-6/ Omega-3 Essential Fatty Acids" explains that "A lower ratio of omega-6/omega-3 fatty acids is more desirable in reducing the risk of many of the chronic diseases of high prevalence in Western societies," including

cardiovascular disease, cancer, and inflammatory and autoimmune diseases.

Ultimately, replacing omega-6 vegetable oils with MUFAs like extra-virgin olive oil and avocado oil while adding in omega-3 rich foods will enhance nutritional balance, leading to a stronger inflammatory defense. The Core Three Plan encourages *three servings of fatty fish per week based on the protein list in the previous chapter*. This provides an average of 375 milligrams of omega-3 fatty acids per day—an amount recommended for optimal health. If you are not a fish eater, fish oil supplements can fill in nutritional gaps. If you're completely animal-free, algae oil supplements are equally suitable. (In fact, the reason fish contain omegas is that they feed on algae!) Either way, always check with your doctor, especially if you are taking any prescription medications, to ensure supplement safety. You will also notice that fish oils are not counted in the Core Three fat list in this chapter. That is because most calories in fish come from proteins that have an anti-inflammatory fat bonus.

**Saturated Fats**

Unlike MUFAs and PUFAs, saturated fats can increase inflammation. That is why the Dietary Guidelines for Americans recommend that no more than 10 percent of total calories come from saturated fats. Based on a 1,600-calorie diet, this equals 160 calories, or about 17 grams per day. Although you need saturated fats for physiological and structural functions, your body can make enough to fulfill this obligation. Dietary saturated fats are mostly sourced from animal fats like red meat, whole-milk dairy, and butter, but they are also found in plant-sourced fats like coconut and palm oil, as well as processed snack foods (cookies, chips, pastries). You can still enjoy saturated fats in your diet, as long as they don't replace more-nutritious anti-inflammatory fats.

**WHAT ABOUT COCONUT OIL AND GHEE?**
Coconut oil is often touted as a "health" food with the potential to fight inflammation, suppress appetite, and burn fat. While studies are mixed on how much of a health food coconut oil is, the fact remains: The lion's share of coconut oil is saturated fat. No matter how you drizzle it, mix it, or pour it, coconut oil can raise LDL cholesterol. It is also unclear whether appetite-suppressing MCT oils are widespread in commercially available coconut oil. Regardless, adding coconut oil into your cooking rotation is a safe practice if you have healthy cholesterol levels, but extra-virgin olive oil still reigns supreme.

Ghee, or clarified butter, is another misleading health food in the wellness industry, with similar claims to coconut oil. Ghee differs from butter in that the milk solids are removed, making it easier to digest. Like coconut oil, it is still primarily saturated fat. Not surprisingly, there is inconclusive evidence to support the health claims. That does not mean you should avoid it or that it's harmful, but it might not have the same positive effects that MUFA-rich extra-virgin olive oil and other anti-inflammatory fats listed in the table provide.

**Trans Fats**
There are a few different types of trans fats—some are found naturally in animal foods like beef and dairy, and others are manufactured. Manufactured, or artificial, trans fats are created by adding hydrogen to liquid vegetable oil, converting it into partially hydrogenated oil. This process turns the oil solid, increases its shelf life, and decreases the chance of spoilage or rancidity. While trans fats originated with margarines and shortenings, the process soon started popping up in fast-food restaurants and commercially produced snack foods like cookies and pastries as companies learned how "useful" it could be. Artificial trans fats, or partially hydrogenated oils, are probably the only type of fat that you'll ever hear a dietitian advise you to completely avoid. Fortunately, the FDA banned them from the US food supply as of January 1, 2020. Why? Studies repeatedly and categorically confirm the dangers of these types of trans fats. They lower HDL cholesterol, raise LDL cholesterol, and significantly increase the risk of heart disease. Cutting them out of our food supply dramatically reduces inflammatory diseases, insulin resistance, and the

risk of heart attack. Yes, there are still trace amounts found naturally in animal foods like beef and cheese, but experts concluded that the risk was much higher when these fats are consumed in manufactured form.

Partially hydrogenated oils should not be confused with fully hydrogenated oils. Fully hydrogenated oils are not considered a trans fat, but they are still pro-inflammatory. They are simply vegetable oils that are turned into solid form through hydrogenation, which makes them more of a saturated fat that is found primarily in ultraprocessed or fried foods. While both types go through a process that turns a liquid oil into a solid form, partially hydrogenated oil is more hazardous to your health than fully hydrogenated oil.

## What Are Age-Fighting Antioxidants?

The term "antioxidants" technically refers more to an activity than to a substance. Nutrients like vitamin C and vitamin E, as well as plant chemicals known as polyphenols, all have antioxidant traits. This means they fight oxidative stress, and thus inflammation, in your body. Oxidative stress is an imbalance of free radicals (unstable atoms) and antioxidants that can cause considerable damage to cells and genetic material.

When you walk outside and breathe in air pollutants or cigarette smoke, it contributes to oxidative stress. When you catch an infection or virus, that's another form of oxidative stress. When you go for a long run, the stress of prolonged exercise on your body can contribute to oxidative stress. Other lifestyle habits—including insufficient sleep, drug and alcohol abuse, and, of course, imbalanced eating habits—can also increase free radical damage that mimics chronic inflammatory contributors.

As you can see, oxidative stress occurs all the time for reasons both in and out of our control, such as simply living and breathing. While some degree of stress is unavoidable, and moderate amounts are perfectly normal, when these stressors pile up over time, stress can take its toll. Not only does excessive free radical exposure accelerate the aging process, but it can also lead to other health conditions, such as cancer, diabetes, heart disease, and kidney diseases.

How can you protect yourself and defend against oxidative stress? I'm glad you asked: a balanced, nutrient-dense diet, of course! The key to unlocking your free radical defense is eating foods that have higher antioxidant activity, along with healthy lifestyle habits consisting of adequate sleep and moderate exercise (which we will discuss in Chapter 8). The best sources include a variety of colorful fruits and vegetables. You don't need to eat every fruit and veggie to benefit—just an assortment of colors will do the trick. Think the rainbow: red apples, orange carrots, yellow squash, green spinach, blueberries, and purple potatoes.

There are tons of additional antioxidants, such as beta-carotene, lycopene, resveratrol, vitamin C, and vitamin E, naturally available in our food supply, and each one is important for various reasons. They also work together, which is why the more diversity, the better. This means you should eat a variety of Core Three foods like fruits, vegetables, whole grains, and anti-inflammatory fats. Specifically, nuts, seeds, avocado, and certain types of oils will create a strong line of defense against oxidative stress.

## How Do Anti-inflammatory Fats Fuel Your Body?

When carbs, your premier fuel source, are not as accessible or are consumed in smaller amounts, your body utilizes fat for energy. The body mobilizes fat cells and converts them into glucose through a not-so-easy-to-pronounce mechanism called gluconeogenesis. Certain types of fats also contribute energy-boosting nutrients that stabilize blood sugars. A study published in the medical journal *PLOS Medicine* in 2016 found that replacing "saturated fat with a diet rich in unsaturated fat, particularly polyunsaturated fat, was beneficial for the regulation of blood sugar."

Adding anti-inflammatory fat to a carb like bread, fruit, crackers, or potatoes can also directly affect how quickly that carb gets broken down. By simply adding more anti-inflammatory fats, you can turn a faster-digesting carb into a much slower-digesting carb, improving insulin and blood sugar harmony. This is due to fat's slower gastric emptying process. Fats remain in your stomach longer, which is also why they add staying power and overall satiety. This is yet another example of why balancing the Core Three macros is critical for energy, appetite, and overall health.

Aside from adding variety, enjoyment, and satisfaction to meals, fats enable absorption of vitamins A, D, E, and K. These vitamins require fat for maximum absorption. Why do we want these vitamins? Well, vitamin A is crucial for eyesight; D supports bone health and immunity and can fight inflammation; E is a powerful antioxidant; and K is important for bones and blood clotting. Fats also provide an energy source and help with cell wall formation.

## What about Blood Lipids?

I have been referencing how *dietary* fats can modulate fats, or lipids, in our blood known as triglycerides and LDL or HDL cholesterol. Blood lipids are fat-like substances found in our blood and body tissues. Lipid levels are routinely under the microscope because high lipid levels raise the risk of heart disease—the leading cause of death in the US—and have zero physical symptoms. You won't know you have high cholesterol until your annual primary care checkup. Statistics show that more than one in ten adults are diagnosed with high cholesterol or high triglycerides each year.

What exactly are HDL and LDL cholesterol? They are lipoproteins, which are proteins that carry fats in your blood, and they can impact your overall health and well-being. Many people get confused about which one is "good" versus "bad." "LDL" stands for "low-density lipoproteins," and "HDL" stands for "high-density lipoproteins." Ultimately, you want more high-density (HDL) than low-density (LDL). I often share the following mnemonic with my clients who have trouble remembering: Think of the L in LDL as "lousy" and the H in HDL as "helpful." Both of these are added together as "total cholesterol." Therefore, if you have high HDL, you will have high total cholesterol.

Like managing your blood cholesterol, managing triglycerides is important for heart health. The reference ranges for blood lipids are as follows:

### LDL (LOUSY CHOLESTEROL)
- Optimal: less than 100 mg/dl
- Acceptable (if you have no other health issues or risk factors): less than 130 mg/dl
- High: greater than 130 mg/dl

### HDL (HELPFUL CHOLESTEROL)
- Optimal: greater than 60 mg/dl
- Acceptable: 41–59 mg/dl
- Low: less than 40 mg/dl

### TRIGLYCERIDES (SHOULD BE TAKEN FASTING)
- Optimal: less than 150 mg/dl
- High: greater than 150 mg/dl

If you have ever seen lab values outside the "optimal" range, don't panic. They don't automatically predict heart disease. Overall susceptibility is measured by an aggregate of various other factors, including family health history, other medical issues like blood pressure, and potentially body fat measurements. Aside from these risk factors, nutrition and exercise can make a significant difference. Studies show a high-fiber, high-anti-inflammatory-fat, minimally processed, and plant-powered diet—all of which is recommended in the Core Three—along with moderate exercise is the ticket for your ticker. The American Heart Association specifically recommends limiting saturated and trans fats while increasing fruits, veggies, whole grains, and fish oils.

What about dietary cholesterol? Common sense would tell you that dietary cholesterol will raise blood cholesterol levels. People often avoid eating cholesterol-rich shrimp for that exact reason. However, most of what disrupts your optimal balance of blood lipids, like LDL and triglycerides, are foods that contain saturated fats, trans fats, and refined sugars. Shrimp is virtually free of saturated fat and, studies show, can increase (helpful) HDL cholesterol with little to no impact on (lousy) LDL cholesterol. Dietary cholesterol is not bad, and blood cholesterol is not all that bad either. Your body can make its own cholesterol in your liver, which is a good thing: Cholesterol helps make cell structures and synthesize hormones and vitamin D.

### The Myth of the Low-Fat Diet

Countless studies demonstrate that moderate-fat diets (those with 30–50 percent total calories from fat) are more effective for weight management and heart health than low-fat diets (those with less than 30 percent total calories from fat). This is quite the opposite of what many diets would lead you to believe. In fact, a 2015 article published in *The Lancet Diabetes & Endocrinology* says that "dietary interventions lower in total fat intake lead to significantly less weight loss compared with higher fat, low-carbohydrate diets." Besides the fact that there is evidence to include fat in your diet if you're trying to avoid weight gain, food is meant to be enjoyed, and fat-rich foods certainly help.

Instead of worrying about high cholesterol, focus on the ratio of HDL to LDL, not just total cholesterol. High LDL is not as detrimental if you also have high HDL. The risk of cardiovascular disease increases based not just on these numbers but also on an accumulation of various circumstances. Overall, it is important to remember that dietary cholesterol does not increase blood cholesterol levels nearly as much as saturated and trans fats, along with fast-digesting refined carbs and sugars. A balanced diet, including plenty of Core Three fiber-rich carbs, lean proteins, and anti-inflammatory fats, plus moderate exercise is your most effective weapon against cardiovascular disease.

## Can I Eat Too Many Fats?

It is possible to eat too much of *any* food or food group, whether that's cookies, chips, avocado, or chicken. When consumed indiscriminately, even vegetables can lead to a variety of unwanted side effects, including gas, bloating, and diarrhea. The real issue is that eating excessive quantities of any food, and feeling out of control about it, is a sign that you're in need of food relationship rehabilitation. You can adjust this mindset, though—start by trying to understand why you're eating more than you need. See Chapter 2 for more on the topic of your relationship with food.

Fat-rich foods are also more calorie-dense than carbs and proteins. For that reason, it can be easier to exceed total calorie and energy needs for the day with a higher-fat diet. This disrupts the benefits of balanced eating. From a medical standpoint, disproportionately high-fat diets can be troublesome for those who have had a gallbladder removed or have a history of gastroparesis. Higher fat intake can also bother those with sensitive tummies and gastrointestinal issues like irritable bowel syndrome or acid reflux. If you do notice digestive distress or are not noticing any substantial weight changes, you can start to reduce your intake.

While there are no fats that are off-limits in Core Three, we want to focus on adding in fats that will have the most profound impact on your overall health and well-being. These types of fats will be listed in the tables that follow for reference.

## Mono- and Polyunsaturated Fats

As explained earlier, certain types of PUFAs, such as peanut, corn, and soybean oils, are higher in omega-6s. If you are concerned with inflammation, you can choose the other listed fats instead. (Each portion listed here is roughly 100 calories and 10 grams of fat.)

| FOOD | FIBER | PORTION |
| --- | --- | --- |
| Almonds | 2g | 12 nuts |
| Avocado | 2g | ⅓ avocado |
| Brazil nuts | 2g | 4 nuts |
| Cashews | 1g | 12 nuts |
| Filberts (hazelnuts) | 1g | 10 nuts |
| Hummus | 3g | ¼ cup |
| Macadamia nuts | 1g | 6 nuts |
| Mayo, reduced fat | 0g | 1 Tbsp. |
| Mayo, regular | 0g | 1 tsp. |
| Nut butters (peanut, almond, cashew) | ~2g | 1 Tbsp. |
| Oils (canola, olive, avocado, peanut, flax) | 0g | 1 Tbsp. |
| Olives | 3g | 15–20 olives |
| Peanuts | 2g | 20 nuts |
| Pecans | 0.5g | 8 halves |
| Pine nuts | 1g | 2 Tbsp. |
| Pistachios | 3g | 32 nuts (2½ Tbsp.) |
| Seeds (chia, hemp, flax, pumpkin, sunflower) | 5–8g | 2 Tbsp. |
| Spread, plant stanol (Benecol), light* | 0g | 2 Tbsp. |
| Spread, plant stanol (Benecol), regular* | 0g | 1 Tbsp. |
| Tahini (sesame paste) | 4g | 1 Tbsp. |
| Walnuts | 1g | 8 halves |

*Benecol butter spread is a particular brand that contains a rich source of plant sterols and stanols, which are exceptionally beneficial for lowering cholesterol. Many other butter spread alternatives are high in processed and pro-inflammatory oils. You are likely better off consuming grass-fed butter or ghee than a processed butter substitute. However, either way, everything is okay in moderation.

## Saturated Fats

These fats can also be enjoyed in moderation but are not considered anti-inflammatory. They can add more variety to your diet while allowing diet flexibility.

| FOOD | FIBER | PORTION |
| --- | --- | --- |
| Butter | 0g | 1 Tbsp. |
| Cacao nibs, raw | 5–9g | 3 Tbsp. |
| Cheese, full-fat or whole-milk (includes cream cheese) | 0g | 1 oz. |
| Coconut, dried, unsweetened, shredded | 2g | 3 Tbsp. |
| Coconut oil | 0g | 1 Tbsp. |
| Ghee | 0g | 1 Tbsp. |
| Yogurt, almond milk, unsweetened | 3–5g | ⅔ cup |
| Yogurt, coconut milk, unsweetened | 2–4g | 1 cup |

Now that we have reviewed the fundamentals of anti-inflammatory fats, you can add them into your diet without fear. Fats like nuts, seeds, avocados, and olive oil are key players in the Core Three: They fuel you while fighting inflammation. Space them throughout the day for maximum benefits and pair them with carbs and proteins for a well-rounded diet. Next, we will discuss how to put everything together for a personalized plan that will help you reach your goals. I will recommend portion suggestions based on your individual needs.

# CHAPTER 7

# Adding In Additional Foods

By now, you may be thinking, "Am I going to feel full and satisfied on this plan?" It is a common concern whenever you try to eat healthier, especially if you're aiming to lose weight. Fortunately, the Core Three Plan is not about deprivation. In fact, this is a rather voluminous diet that would look like a generous amount of food if it were all laid on a table. In addition to the major Core Three macronutrients you've already learned about, there is one critical category of food in the Core Three that is not considered a high-fiber carbohydrate, lean protein, or anti-inflammatory fat: non-starchy veggies. Non-starchy veggies are the foundation of your Core Three diet. They add bulk and provide vital nutrients that support health and weight loss.

Plus, you can spice up your daily menu, get creative, and introduce additional foods that can act as lower-carb alternatives in your favorite meals, such as sandwiches, pastas, noodles, and rice. Familiarizing yourself with all these additional foods will get your healthy eating habits off the ground.

In this chapter, we will review these additional foods to enhance your success on the Core Three Healthy Eating Plan. You will understand which vegetables are considered non-starchy and how they play a vital role, not just for weight loss but for overall health. I will also provide low-carb alternatives that don't count as a carb but can offer similar satisfaction. Finally, I will explain how condiments and sweeteners can fit in so that you can enjoy everything you're eating with plenty of flavor.

## Non-Starchy Veggies Are Vital

Non-starchy veggies are significantly lower in carbohydrates compared with starchy veggies like potatoes, beans, peas, and corn. For example, 1 cup of white potatoes has around 26 grams of carbohydrates, while 1 cup of broccoli has about 6 grams of carbs. After subtracting the 2 grams of fiber from this 6-gram count, you are left with only 4 grams of net carbs. Non-starchy veggies not only supply fiber, helping you reach your daily quota, but are also teeming with micronutrients like potassium, iron, magnesium, and vitamin C; antioxidants; and water.

Considering the volume and nutrients you obtain for such low carb content, the Core Three Plan encourages AT LEAST three servings of non-starchy veggies per day (as outlined in the table that follows). As long as you account for what else you eat with them, non-starchy veggies can be incorporated freely. The only exception to eating these plant foods ad infinitum is if you deal with digestion issues or have a special condition, some of which are discussed in Chapter 10.

The Non-Starchy Vegetables table includes mostly fresh vegetables, but you can also enjoy frozen and canned versions. Frozen vegetables can be more nutritious than fresh because they're flash frozen as they're harvested—this process preserves and locks in nutrients. Fresh veggies lose their nutrient quality as they ripen and age. Canned veggies—considered a type of cooked veggie—also have plenty to offer, including fiber and antioxidants, although they tend to be much higher in sodium. If you have a history of high blood pressure, it is best to limit anything canned or opt for versions labeled "low-sodium."

## Non-Starchy Vegetables

A serving is 1 cup raw or ½ cup cooked. Fiber is based on 1 cup raw.

| FOOD | FIBER |
|------|-------|
| Artichokes | 2.5g |
| Artichoke hearts | 13g |
| Asparagus | 3g |
| Baby corn | 4g |
| Bamboo shoots | 3g |
| Bean sprouts | 2g |
| Beans (green, wax, Italian) | 3g |
| Beets | 4g |
| Broccoli | 2g |
| Broccoli slaw, packaged, no dressing | 4g |
| Brussels sprouts | 3g |
| Cabbage | 2g |
| Carrots | 4g |
| Cauliflower | 4g |
| Celery | 2g |
| Chayote | 2g |
| Coleslaw, packaged, no dressing | 2g |
| Cucumber | 1g |
| Daikon | 2g |
| Eggplant | 2g |
| Fennel | 3g |
| Gourds (bitter, bottle, luffa, bitter melon) | 3g |
| Greens (arugula, collard, dandelion, mustard, purslane, turnip) | 2g |

| FOOD | FIBER |
|------|-------|
| Hearts of palm | 3.5g |
| Jicama | 6g |
| Kale | 1g |
| Kohlrabi | 5g |
| Leeks | 2g |
| Mushrooms | 1g |
| Okra | 3g |
| Onions | 3g |
| Pea pods | 1.5g |
| Peppers (green, red, yellow, orange) | 3g |
| Radishes | 2g |
| Rutabaga | 3g |
| Sauerkraut (good source of probiotics but high in sodium) | 4g |
| Scallions (aka green onions) | 3g |
| Spinach | 1g |
| Squash, summer (yellow, zucchini) | 1g |
| Sugar snap peas | 2g |
| Swiss chard | 1g |
| Tomato | 2g |
| Tomato sauce, unsweetened, canned | 4g |
| Tomato/vegetable juice | 2g |
| Turnips | 2g |
| Water chestnuts | 6g |

## Low-Carb Alternatives

We know that deprivation does not create a healthy relationship with food or long-term success with any plan. For that reason, every carbohydrate food has a non-carbohydrate alternative. These options help prevent the proverbial "diet burnout" that comes from repeatedly eating the same foods.

## Explaining the Exchange

Since these are *alternatives* to carbs, they consist mostly of proteins and fats. Next to each food, you will see how it translates into a protein and/or fat serving. This allows easy macronutrient tracking.

### Cereal Alternatives

| FOOD | FIBER | PORTION | EXCHANGE |
| --- | --- | --- | --- |
| Catalina Crunch | 9g | ½ cup | ½ fat + ½ protein |
| Homemade Cinnamon Nut Granola (see Chapter 13) | 4g | ¼ cup | 1 fat |
| Julian Bakery ProGranola | 12g | ½ cup | ½ fat + ½ protein |
| Magic Spoon Cereal (Cocoa, Fruity, Cinnamon) | 1–2g | ¾ cup | ½ fat + ½ protein |

### Bread Alternatives

| FOOD | FIBER | PORTION | EXCHANGE |
| --- | --- | --- | --- |
| DIY Gluten-Free Bagel (see Chapter 13) | 4g | 1 bagel | 1 fat |
| Julian Bakery Paleo Thin Bread (almond or seed medley) | 10–12g | 2 slices | 1 fat + ½ protein |
| SOLA Bread (golden wheat) | 8g | 2 slices | 1 fat |
| Low Carb, Whole Wheat Tortilla, La Tortilla Factory | 16g | 2 tortillas | ½ protein |
| Tortilla, Mama Lupe's Low Carb | 8g | 2 tortillas | ½ protein |
| Tortilla, Tumaro's Carb Wise White Protein Wrap | 6g | 1 tortilla | ½ protein |

## Pasta/Noodle Alternatives

| FOOD | FIBER | PORTION | EXCHANGE |
|---|---|---|---|
| Palmini | 5g | 1½ cups | Non-starchy veg |
| Shirataki (konjac) noodles | 2g | 4 oz. | Non-starchy veg |
| Spiralized zucchini (aka zoodles) | 2g | 1 cup cooked | 0 |

## Cracker Alternatives

| FOOD | FIBER | PORTION | EXCHANGE |
|---|---|---|---|
| Flackers | 8g | 8 crackers | 1 fat |
| GG Scandinavian Fiber Crispbread | 16g | 4 crackers | 0 |
| Mary's Gone Crackers (gluten-free) | 2g | 8 crackers | ½ fat + ½ carb |

## Sweeteners

If you prefer sweet-tasting foods and beverages, you must work with this proclivity, not against it. Sweetening foods is not an "unhealthy behavior"—it just depends on what type of sweeteners you're using, how much you're using, and how often you're adding them in. There are plenty of options to satisfy an urge for a sugar surge.

### Artificial Sweeteners

Artificial sweeteners like aspartame (Equal), saccharin (Sweet'N Low), sucralose (Splenda), and plant-based stevia are zero-calorie chemical sweeteners intended to keep sugar and blood glucose levels in check. But are they really helping you achieve your goals? Studies show artificial sweeteners might actually spark appetite and create hunger in certain individuals. A 2013 review published in *Diabetes Care* discovered that sucralose (Splenda) ingestion increased blood glucose and insulin secretion rate. Why? One explanation is that when you eat something *sweet,* whether from zero-calorie sweeteners or refined table sugar, your brain discerns the taste and prepares for an anticipated blood sugar surge. This signals your pancreas to dispatch insulin to retrieve sugar from your blood. When insulin finds out that it was all a ruse, it remains elevated, demanding what it was originally promised: sugar. Choosing Splenda over refined sugar might feel like the smart move, but it might also be why you can't stop snacking on sweets after dinner.

Of course, quantity matters. It is fine to include sweeteners in your diet in moderation, which I classify as less than two packets per day. One packet in your coffee each day will have minimal impact. However, artificial sweeteners can easily add up. If you start your day with a cup of Splenda-sweetened coffee and then eat a sugar-free yogurt and grab a protein bar on the way out the door, that is three to four packets right there. When lunchtime arrives, if you guzzle down an aspartame-sweetened diet tea with your salad and then pop a piece of sugar-free mint gum, that's another two to three packets. This would explain why you're anxiously craving sweets by early afternoon. Sure, there are other reasons why this could be happening, but if cutting down on something that has zero nutritional value may help, it is certainly worth a try.

## The Diet Soda Dilemma

As with artificial sweeteners, diet soda provides little to no nutritional value. It is often used as a method to cut calories, satisfy a sugar craving, or get a caffeine boost. While it may contain zero calories and no sugar, that does not mean it has zero effect on your body. Most diet sodas are full of artificial sweeteners that can increase blood sugars and appetite while destroying healthy gut bacteria. Diet soda can even be linked to weight gain, not weight loss.

### The Effects of Artificial Sweeteners on the Body

While there are claims that artificial sweeteners can cause diseases, scientific evidence has not supported that. First, "it is the position of the Academy of Nutrition and Dietetics that consumers can *safely* enjoy a range of nutritive and nonnutritive sweeteners." Second, the National Cancer Institute reassures us that "studies of...FDA-approved sweeteners have not demonstrated clear evidence of an association with cancer in humans." There is evidence, however, that nonnutritive sweeteners can interfere with the gut microbiome. A 2018 study published in the journal *Molecules*, titled "Measuring Artificial Sweeteners Toxicity Using a Bioluminescent Bacterial Panel," explains that once ingested, sweeteners like aspartame and sucralose destroy healthy gut bacteria that support vital bodily functions, including one's immune system and metabolism.

Of course, if it's an occasional treat and you're meeting your other health goals, there is little to no harm done from drinking a diet soda. If soda is a frequent beverage choice, ask yourself, "Why am I choosing soda over water or any other type of drink?" Is it a mechanism to suppress appetite or satisfy a sweet tooth? Are you in need of an energy boost, or are you simply someone who enjoys a bubbly beverage?

If you're developing a dependency on diet soda, however, it is time to reduce your consumption. Try naturally infused seltzer or sparkling water with a splash of juice. There are also several brands that use natural sweeteners and offer the same fizzy satisfaction with few calories and little sugar. Examples include Spindrift, OLI-POP, Bubly, Sipp, and Zevia (sweetened with plant-based stevia).

## Natural Sweeteners

Overall, if you rely on artificial sweeteners for taste, consider trying alternatives such as cinnamon, vanilla extract, and even fresh fruit to add more natural flavor instead. Plant-derived sweeteners like stevia and monk fruit are also sweet and may prove to be a better option than chemical versions. Some studies show stevia may improve blood sugar and insulin homeostasis, although more research is needed on this topic.

If you prefer the natural flavor of real sugar, honey, or syrup, those are acceptable in moderation as well. Understand that these types of sweeteners can also increase blood sugars and insulin levels, contributing to roller-coaster energy levels, reactive sweet cravings, and weight gain over time. Does this mean drizzling some honey into your yogurt or mixing one sugar packet into your coffee is a problem? No. It's just important to be mindful of how quickly these added sugars can tally up. In the recipe chapters, you will see that I include honey or syrup in a few of the recipes as an optional sweetener. This gives you an idea of how it can be healthily incorporated.

Remember to keep all added sugar, such as from sugar packets, honey, agave, and other syrups, in your daily flexible carb calories. A flexible carb is about 100 calories, which is equivalent to about 5 teaspoons of honey, agave, or syrup. This table gives you a few ideas for how to add flavor without excess sugar.

## Sweeten and Lighten

Using only the amount listed in the table does not count toward any particular macro.

| SWEETENER/LIGHTENER | PORTION |
| --- | --- |
| Cinnamon | 1–3 tsp. |
| Flavored creamers | 1–2 Tbsp. |
| Half-and-half | 1 oz. |
| Honey | 1–2 tsp. |
| Milk | ½ cup or less |
| nutpods | 3–4 Tbsp. |
| Silk Almond Creamer | 2–3 Tbsp. |
| Silk Oatmilk Creamer | 1–2 Tbsp. |
| Stevia or monk fruit | 1–2 packets per day |
| Traditional sugar (white, brown, or in the raw) | ½–1 packet per day |
| Vanilla extract | 1–2 tsp. |

## Condiments

Sauces, dips, and spreads add calories, salt, and sugar to your diet. However, if they make certain foods like veggies or proteins more appealing, condiments can be worth it, depending on the nutritional profile and frequency of use. If the condiment has more than 5 grams of sugar or 5 grams of saturated fat per 2 tablespoons, use it sparingly (2- to 3-tablespoon portions at a time). Otherwise, using seasonings (like fresh herbs garlic, onions, and black pepper) and anti-inflammatory fats (like olive oil, avocado, mayo, and hummus) can add plenty of flavor. Refer to the recipes in Chapters 13–15 for additional ideas and alternative taste-enhancing methods. Otherwise, here are some basic condiments you can enjoy regularly that will not count toward any macro category:

## Flexible Core Three Condiments

Using only the amount listed in the table does not count toward any particular macro.

| CONDIMENT | PORTION |
|---|---|
| Coconut aminos | |
| Hot sauce | |
| Low-sodium soy sauce | |
| Mustard (regular, stone ground, Dijon, spicy, horseradish) | |
| Salad dressing (See recipes in Chapters 14–15 for DIY salad dressings you can make at home.) | <50 calories per 2 Tbsp. |
| Salsa (green or red; mild, medium, or spicy) | |
| Seasonings (pepper, oregano, garlic, onion powder, cinnamon, nutmeg, turmeric, basil, parsley, chives, sesame seeds, cumin, thyme, dill, ginger, paprika, etc.) | |
| Sriracha | |
| Taco sauce (mild, medium, or spicy) | |
| Teriyaki sauce | 3 Tbsp. or less = 0 carbs<br>4–6 Tbsp. = 1 carb |
| Tomato sauce, jarred, store-brought | ½ cup or less = 0 carbs<br>>½ cup–1 cup = 1 carb<br>>1 cup–2 cups = 2 carbs |
| Vinegar (apple cider, balsamic, red wine, white, etc.) | |

Rigid diet plans rarely work for the long term. Structured plans that offer variety and flexibility—like Core Three—are the most effective, sustainable solution to finding your healthiest, happiest weight. The additional foods discussed in this chapter will make a major difference in how satisfied you feel with your food choices, so there is no deprivation. But what would a healthy eating plan be without including some type of movement? In the next chapter, I'll explain where exercise fits in and the best way to get your body moving.

# CHAPTER 8

# Exercise—a Reward, Not a Punishment

Nutrition and exercise go hand in hand, especially when it comes to your health. Still, there is a lot of contradictory information regarding how much, how often, and what types of exercise are best. Some believe that exercise is not necessary at all to finding your happiest "you" weight, declaring that it's diet over dumbbells. Others become attached to their cardio machines, trying to melt away as much body fat as possible. Either way, if the balance is broken, so is a chance at a healthy relationship with exercise. My recommendation: Moderate exercise is the best way to *feel good in your body*—a primary Core Three Plan objective.

In this chapter, I'll outline the benefits of exercise. I will also provide clear exercise recommendations and explain why it is important to combine a variety of movements, from cardio to strength training. For those with more active lifestyles beyond the Core Three exercise recommendations, you'll find guidelines on how to adjust the meal plan for additional nutrient needs. We'll also take a look at your relationship with exercise and how to overcome the all-or-nothing attitude so that you can sustain your success. Finally, we will talk about why increasing exercise is not the only way to find your healthiest, happiest weight.

## The Benefits of Exercise

The benefits of exercise are endless. The irony is that most people feel like they need a reward *after* they exercise, potentially undoing its benefits. If that describes you, try to shift your mindset and think of exercise as a reward in itself; it can help improve your relationship with your body and with food. For some, like Erratic Eaters and Dependent Eaters, exercising mindfully is particularly beneficial. You don't need fancy equipment to reap the rewards, which include:

- **Better mood:** Exercise releases feel-good neurotransmitters known as endorphins.
- **Increased energy:** Physical activity circulates oxygen and nutrients to your tissues that helps your cardiovascular system work more efficiently.
- **Improved sleep:** Regular exercise can realign your internal body clock or natural circadian rhythm.
- **Easier digestion:** Exercise strengthens the muscles and reduces the blood flow to the intestines in your digestive tract, which helps regulate bowel movements. Studies also show that exercise can improve the microbiome and balance of healthy gut bacteria.
- **Stronger immune system:** Physical activity can directly modulate the immune system by promoting the release of anti-inflammatory cytokines and circulating lymphocytes and enabling immune cell recruitment. Studies show

moderate exercise can lower the incidence and intensity of viral infections.
- **Manageable appetite:** Aerobic exercise like running, walking, and cycling can help regulate appetite due to its suppression of hormones that drive hunger, particularly one called ghrelin.
- **Harmonized cortisol and stress levels:** Moderate exercise can help regulate stress levels and hormones, helping you feel more relaxed and emotionally stable.
- **Enhanced insulin function:** Exercise, especially strength training, improves insulin function and stabilizes blood sugars.
- **Healthier heart:** Physical activity increases HDL (healthy cholesterol) and reduces triglycerides, protecting against cardiovascular disease.
- **Fewer injuries:** Exercise improves bone mass and density and fights age-related muscle loss. This diminishes wear and tear in connective tissues.
- **Improved body image:** Focusing on building lean muscle and noticing improvements can positively alter how you feel about the way you look.

## The Core Three Way to Exercise

There is no perfect amount of exercise, because it always depends on the individual, but having a goal can help. The Core Three recommends a realistic 3 hours of moderate-intensity activity per week, including a combination of cardio and strength training exercises. This can be divided up however you like, whether it's 1 hour for 3 days, 45 minutes for 4 days, or 30 minutes for up to 6 days per week. This recommendation is in line with a 2012 study published in the *American Journal of Physiology*, which revealed that simply exercising for 30 minutes per day is just as effective for weight loss, and beneficial for health, as a full hour. It is also important that you combine cardio, strength training, and restorative movement—this is the best complement to the Core Three Healthy Eating Plan.

### Cardiovascular Exercise

Cardio is any movement that raises your breathing and heart rate for a sustained time period (10 minutes or more). If you are someone who craves the endorphin boost after a cycling class, run at the park, or refreshing swim in the pool, it's no surprise. Endorphins lift your spirits, spark creativity, and clear your mind. Of the three total recommended Core Three exercise hours per week, you can *aim for 1–2 hours per week of cardio* like jogging, brisk walking, cycling, hiking, or swimming.

### MORE ON EXERCISE INTENSITY LEVELS

Although I recommend moderate exercise because I believe for many it's easier to sustain, vigorous exercise can be more effective when you are strapped for time. Light exercise is also beneficial, as it allows more

mindfulness. The easiest way to measure the intensity of exercise (light, moderate, or vigorous) is the "talk test":

- Light intensity allows for a full conversation and even singing.
- Moderate intensity means you can talk but not sing.
- Vigorous or strenuous exercise allows only a few words before you have to pause to breathe, as in running, swimming, and heavier weightlifting.

## Types of Exercise

Fortunately, there are so many different options to log your exercise hours, whether in the form of cardio or strength training. You don't have to do them all, you just have to find a few that work for you. Here are some ideas to get you started.

### Walking

If you're not sure where to start, walking is incredibly underrated. A 2015 review conducted by Norwich Medical School and published in the *British Journal of Sports Medicine* found that subjects who adhered to consistent and routine walking demonstrated a significant reduction in blood pressure and body fat, a slowed resting heart rate, lowered cholesterol, and improved depression scores with better quality of life. You don't have to overexert yourself to clock in your cardio.

### High-Intensity Interval Training

High-intensity interval training (HIIT) is another effective option. This is an activity that alternates among light, moderate, and vigorous exercise. You push yourself hard for a short period of time, such as 1–2 minutes, and follow with a few minutes of light or moderate activity. An example of HIIT cardio is walking for 3–5 minutes and then running for 1–3 minutes and continuing this cycle several times. HIIT can accelerate fat-burning and help you feel empowered at the same time.

### Resistance Training

Resistance training is not limited to weightlifting—it is any movement that involves pressing or pulling against a force. The main outcome is an increase in strength and muscle, both of which are important for weight loss and better body image. Whenever you lose weight, you may lose some muscle. While muscle loss is unavoidable, you can mitigate it by increasing resistance exercise. Your body also naturally starts losing muscle around age forty, and that continues through the second half of life. Whether you're losing muscle from age or weight loss, the end result is a slower metabolism and increased insulin resistance.

*Of the total 3 hours per week recommended, aim for 60–90 minutes per week of moderate resistance training.* Resistance training includes lifting dumbbells, using machines or resistance bands, or simply using your own body weight through push-ups and wall presses. The stronger you become, the more empowered you will feel.

### Mindful and Meditative Movement

Moving mindfully involves sensory awareness and paying attention to how you physically feel—without judgment or reacting—with a special focus on breathing. Tuning in to your breathing strengthens the mind-body connection. A mind-body connection means feeling like you are in touch with the signs, symptoms, and signals your body consistently, naturally, and deliberately communicates. The best part is that practicing more mindfulness in other areas of life can help you naturally become a more mindful eater: You eventually grow more aware of physiological hunger and fullness cues. Erratic and Dependent Eaters can benefit from mindfulness because it improves self-regulation and the ability to lead your own thoughts, emotions, and behaviors.

Mindful and meditative movement can be incorporated into any of the following activities:

- Yoga
- Light walking
- Stretching
- Bicycling
- Kayaking or canoeing
- Swimming
- Dancing

- Pilates
- Tai chi

You can really take any type of activity and make it more mindful, and therefore gratifying, by asking yourself these five questions:

1. How do I feel: energized or tired?
2. How does it feel to move my body this way or that way?
3. What muscles do I feel activated during this particular movement?
4. Are my muscles achy and exhausted or engaged and energized?
5. Do I feel stronger than the last time I did this exercise?

Mindful and meditative exercise can help foster a healthier relationship with food and improved well-being. Researchers from the University of Florida performed a study in 2018 on seventy-five women between the ages of eighteen and thirty. They were randomly assigned either to twice-weekly yoga classes for 12 weeks or to a control condition with no exercise. The women doing yoga practiced breathing techniques, meditation, and active poses. After completion, the women who had practiced yoga reported improvement in body image, less body dissatisfaction, and a more positive view of their appearance.

No matter what type of activity you choose, make it more mindful by engaging your senses, focusing on deep breathing, and getting rid of self-judgments. Don't worry about how you look, whether you're doing the movement perfectly, or the outcome. Just be.

## Adjusting the Core Three Healthy Eating Plan for Exercise

If you exercise 3 hours per week or are working on increasing your total, there is no need to change the eating plan to accommodate activity levels. The plan supports a weekly 3 hours.

However, if you are an avid exerciser, participating much more than 3 hours per week, you may need to add to the plan. Undereating can exacerbate muscle loss, increase chances of burnout, and potentially lead to injury. First, make sure your urge to exercise is well intentioned and not distorted or unhealthy. If you simply enjoy it, are training for an event, or are a professional, then you will need to make the following adjustments to your eating plan:

- If you're exercising 4–6 hours per week, add in one additional carb, protein, and fat serving to your plan. For example, if you are following a 4-carb, 4-protein, and 4-fat-per-day plan, then you would now consume a minimum of 5 carbs per day, along with 5 proteins and 5 fats. In Chapter 9, I will explain how you can further personalize in case this feels like too much or too little food.

- If you're exercising more than 6 hours per week, add in another portion—or two total—of each macro category. For example, if you were following a 4-carb-per-day plan, increase that to a minimum of 6 carbs, 6 proteins, and 6 fats. Pay attention to how you feel to determine if you need more or less after 3 weeks.

### The Best Time to Exercise

The best time to exercise is when you have the most energy. Some experts believe exercise is more productive in the morning, as it helps set the tone for the day. While this may be true, not everyone is a morning person. Further, if waking up to exercise means sleeping fewer hours, it can do more harm than good. No matter what, when you exercise is up to you and must be sustainable for lasting results.

Flexible carbs can remain at one to two servings per day, regardless of activity level. Make sure to stay hydrated, especially on exercise days, potentially drinking 3 liters (101 ounces) per day. Always pay attention to the color of your urine to gauge hydration status. If you're exercising more than 4–5 hours per week, you might need to add electrolytes to your water like sodium, potassium, magnesium, and chloride,

which can all be lost through intense exercise and heavy sweating. (You can find more information about hydration in Chapter 3.)

Give the meal plan 3 weeks to determine if you want to cut back down on portions, but remember, to sustain a highly active lifestyle, you will need adequate fuel. If your goal is simply to lose weight and burn body fat, 3 hours per week is easy to sustain and conducive for well-being.

## Timed Eating for Exercise

On days that you plan for activity, adjust your eating schedule for proper energy and recovery.

### Eating Before You Exercise

If you exercise when you wake up, you can do so on an empty stomach, if you feel okay. If you notice that your workouts significantly improve when you have eaten, especially if you feel dizzy or lack energy when you don't eat, adjust your plan. Choose food that's more carb-based and easy to digest, such as:

- A banana (1 carb)
- A slice of toast with 1 tablespoon of peanut butter (1 carb + 1 fat)
- ⅔ cup of dry Cheerios (1 carb)

If you exercise later in the day, exercise right before a meal, 2–3 hours after a meal, or 1 hour after a lighter snack. You need to allow your body time to properly digest and metabolize the meal so that it's converted into fuel and doesn't lead to a stomachache.

### Eating After You Exercise

Post-workout meal planning is also important, especially if you were already hungry beforehand. Balancing food groups and including a carbohydrate, protein, and fat helps your body fully recover. Eating within 2 hours after your workout may help boost muscle growth and regulate your appetite later on.

If you're exercising more intensely and for longer than 60 minutes, you might need to plan a bit more carefully. The International Society of Sports Nutrition recommends consuming a high-quality protein within 2 hours after exercise and every 3–4 hours for the best muscle protein synthesis rates, body composition, and performance. If it's not time for a meal, you're pressed for time, or you don't have much appetite, a snack can suffice. Ideal recovery snacks include a combination of protein and carbohydrates, such as:

- 6 ounces Greek yogurt (1 protein) and ⅔ cup cereal (1 carb)
- 2 ounces reduced-fat cheese (1 protein) with 1 ounce crackers (1 carb)
- 2 eggs (½ protein) with 1 slice of toast (1 carb)
- good! Snacks Protein Bar (1 protein + 1 carb + ½ fat)

- OWYN ready-to-drink shake (weight management) (1 protein + 1½ carbs + 1 fat)

Maximize your exercise by properly eating for recovery, energy, and muscle growth.

## How Is Your Relationship with Exercise?

If you have an unhealthy relationship with your body or food, chances are your relationship with exercise suffers as well. Is exercise a form of punishment, compensation for food you ate, or something that you must do regardless of how tired you are? Do you cancel plans to exercise or spend a good chunk of your paycheck on classes, apps, or exercise machines? Or conversely, do you dread exercise or find it overwhelming? Does the idea of exercise transport you back to the days of middle school when you would find any excuse to skip gym class? If so, it's likely that your relationship with exercise needs some patching up.

If you think you might have a dysfunctional relationship with exercise, let's delve a bit deeper. Does it have to do with worries of weight gain or a need to feel in control? Or does it make you feel good and productive? On the contrary, are you afraid of failing before you even try? Are you convinced that you won't enjoy exercise or will even experience discomfort or pain? Do you trust that exercise will actually make you feel better, not worse? You need to have a healthy relationship with exercise to find your happy medium. It's important to embrace it—without abusing it—for optimal physical and mental well-being.

### Overcoming the All-or-Nothing

You don't need to exercise every day to find your happiest, healthiest weight. Finding a happy medium, like the Core Three's recommended 3 hours per week, is the secret formula to sticking with an effective exercise routine that makes you feel empowered and supports a healthy relationship with your body and food. Drop the all-or-nothing and replace it with *whenever possible*. Overcome the all-or-nothing and just MOVE:

- **M—Make it sociable.** If you're more of a social butterfly, reach out to your friends, family, or colleagues to do it together.
- **O—Obtain accountability.** We always perform better when we to take ownership of our actions. Keep track of your exercise in a journal, sign up for a series of classes, invest in a trainer, commit to meeting a friend, or register for a marathon or charity walk/run.
- **V—Vary it up to find something you love.** Keep trying new forms of exercise until you find one that works. You're more likely to stick with it when it's enjoyable.

- **E—Ease into it.** Start slow and small. Even 1 day per week, or 10 minutes per day, is better than nothing.

## The Truth about Exercise and Weight Loss

Exercise can help you lose weight, but that does not mean it should be the only reason you make the commitment. In fact, it's often best to take weight loss out of the equation and instead focus on non-scale wins like improved energy, better digestion, disease prevention, and an uplifted mood. Yet most people attribute weight loss as the motivator to lace up their sneakers. According to a 2013–2016 survey conducted by the CDC, 62.9 percent of adults who reported trying to lose weight were doing so through exercise. Understandably, if your goal is to shed pounds, it makes sense to think walking, running, or swimming will get you there.

However, a 2007 review published by the *Journal of the American Dietetic Association* found that subjects who participated in weight loss–focused randomized clinical trials had minimal to no weight loss through exercise alone. Combining a "reduced-energy [lower calorie] diet and exercise" had the best results and increased probability for weight loss maintenance. The bottom line: Exercise alone is not the ticket to surefire weight loss. Why doesn't exercise produce weight loss when it burns calories and energy? There are several possibilities as to why sweating it out doesn't directly lead to slimming down:

- **You are overestimating calories burned.** Exercise does burn calories, but not as many as you may think. Only an average of 15 percent of total calories burned comes from additional planned exercise. However, if you are hyperfocused on the calories you're burning in a class or cardio session, it may subconsciously lead to the desire to eat more later. Do not think of exercise as a means of burning calories, but rather as a method to boost energy and relieve stress.
- **You want to reward yourself with food.** It is understandable you want to reward yourself for hard work. Unfortunately, food is often the most convenient reward, undoing your hard work. Find nonfood alternatives to incentivize your efforts, like meeting or calling a friend afterward. If you hit certain milestones, like exercising consistently for 2 months straight, you can splurge on a new bag, concert tickets, or a restorative massage. Don't forget: The real reward is exercise itself.
- **Your body may be stressed.** Exercise is a type of stress on the body—a good stress, but a stress nonetheless. While moderate exercise is an effective stress manager, intense exercise elevates cortisol (the stress hormone). A 2011 study published in *Psychoneuroendocrinology* suggests that "repeated physical stress of intensive training and competitive races is associated with elevated cortisol exposure over prolonged periods of time." Research conducted by University College London in 2017 discovered that cortisol levels positively correlated with weight and body fat. In other words, high cortisol levels are often detected in individuals who have higher body fat accumulation—this suggests that excess cortisol can lead to excess weight gain. The same can happen with any type of repeated or chronic stress.

While exercise may help with weight loss, do not overdo it. Overexercising can make it harder to focus on the Core Three Healthy Eating Plan. Exercise at your own pace and find activities that are sustainable.

There is no denying that exercise, including cardio, strength training, and mindful movement, offers benefits. When done in moderation, along with a balanced eating plan, exercise makes you feel better. Feeling better will motivate you to take care of your health. That's how eating and exercise work in tandem. Empower and motivate yourself by viewing exercise as a reward and not as a punishment for eating. In the next chapter, we will discuss how to continue setting yourself up to succeed by further personalizing the Core Three Plan.

# 3 PERSONALIZING AND SUSTAINING THE PLAN

# CHAPTER 9

# Personalizing the Plan

When it comes to your diet, get personal. Just as you have personal needs and preferences, you cannot expect to eat the same way as everyone else—everyone's nutritional needs vary. The Core Three Plan provides the foundation for healthy eating, and the personalization is what builds the framework. Personalization will allow you to make room for your favorite foods and beverages, like alcohol and caffeine, while still meeting your nutritional goals. Taking all these factors into consideration will allow you to be successful, sustain results, and prevent burnout.

In this chapter, I will explain how you can further customize this plan for weight loss goals based on your response and results. We will touch upon supplements and how they could fill in nutritional gaps. I will explain what a flexible carb is and why it can be vital for finding more food freedom. We will also discuss how alcohol and caffeine fit into the picture to avoid feelings of deprivation.

## Personalizing the Plan

Typically, the way you eat to achieve your goals is the way you must eat to sustain results as well. Yet, as you progress, you may need to adjust to keep the momentum going. Let's look at some common scenarios and how you can adjust Core Three to meet those needs.

### Personalizing the Plan to Accelerate Weight Loss

Initially, you were following the Core Three formula to determine how many portions of carbs, proteins, and fats to eat for the day. You may have also added in more servings based on your activity or exercise regimen. If after *three* weeks you do not notice any changes—I'm not just talking about the number on the scale—in body fat percentage, the fit of your clothes, or how you feel, you can adjust in a few ways:

- **Lower your macro servings.** If you're eating five servings of each macro, you can adjust down to four servings of each macro. If you're eating four serving of each macro, you can adjust down to three servings. This is also particularly helpful if you have entered a new weight category. If you started the plan at 165 pounds and four servings of each macro and are now 145 pounds, you will likely need to adjust down to three servings based on the weight changes. Lowering macro servings will work only if you started at four servings or higher per day. Eating fewer than three servings of each can be too restrictive, unhealthy, and unsustainable and may backfire later. If you're already at three servings per day, consider the rest of these adjustments.

- **Restructure eating timing.** Another option is to eat your carbohydrate servings earlier in the day—at breakfast, lunch, and/or snack—and stick with only lean protein, fats, and high-fiber veggies at dinner. This may support better blood sugar and insulin regulation to promote more fat-burning. Please note that this recommendation could lead to after-dinner cravings, as your body still might need that carb at dinner. If so, it's better for your sleep and digestion to have a carb with dinner instead of having an increased urge to eat right before bed.

- **Reduce flexible carbs and meals.** If you're still at a standstill, you can stop using a flexible carb (this will be discussed later) and potentially a flexible meal.

Whatever method you choose, patience is important. Wait *three* weeks before moving on to additional adjustments. Understand that no matter what you do, results happen only when there is consistency.

## Personalizing the Plan to Prevent Discomfort

If you are feeling weak or tired or noticing increased cravings, hunger, or thoughts about food, you may also need to adjust. *Add in one additional carb, fat, and protein serving, and if it doesn't improve, consider eating unlimited portions of lean proteins and anti-inflammatory fats.* While some of you can start with a more structured plan, not everyone responds well to any type of portioning—even if it's not restrictive. Eating unlimited lean proteins and anti-inflammatory fats most effectively aligns with food freedom while making room to listen to your body above all else.

As you lose weight, your body goes through changes. One of those changes could be a slower metabolism. If you're eating less and weighing less, your body requires less energy and fewer calories. Regardless, recognize that if you start to feel deprived or stressed around food, it is no longer healthy to be cutting from your diet.

## Personalizing the Plan for Healthy Weight Maintenance

As you start to notice progress, it is important to set yourself up for sustainability. How? Utilize all the tips and tools in Chapter 11, such as staying accountable with food journaling and body composition analysis as well as securing a strong support system. Other than that, you can slowly liberalize the plan, especially if you want more food freedom in the future.

Around the 3-month mark, or whenever you feel ready, start by only paying attention to carbs. Eat lean protein and anti-inflammatory fats more freely in your diet by trusting your body to guide your choices, and by paying attention to hunger and fullness cues.

If you're still feeling great, then you can stop portioning carbs as well. Continue to prioritize high-fiber carbs, lean proteins, and anti-inflammatory fats; listen to hunger and fullness cues; and practice mindful eating. Later in this chapter, I will address how to include flexible carbs and meals. If, after *three* weeks, all is well, continue healing your relationship with food and your body.

What happens if you notice rebound weight gain? Truthfully, it depends. Is it because you were traveling a lot, eating more than usual during a holiday season, or more stressed than usual? That is just a temporary circumstance and not necessarily a future forecast—don't panic. First, reflect and address these issues. After that, you always have the option to go back to the original formula or start slowly by just portioning out carbs to help manage cravings, and encourage eating enough protein and fats. Not eating enough of these two food groups can be part of the culprit behind overeating.

Always be prepared that there may be times you have a lot going on to prevent you from staying completely aware and mindful. Under these circumstances, your weight may creep up, and your clothes may get tighter. This is normal, and fluctuations of around 3–5 pounds will happen. Don't be alarmed. Simply be patient and self-compassionate before you take action. This plan is here, but must adapt to fit your life for successful weight maintenance.

## Treat Yourself with a Flexible Carb and a Flexible Meal!

It is critical that you give yourself permission to enjoy all the foods you love for success and to sustain the plan. That is where flexible carbs come in. Here is how they work:

- If you weigh less than 200 pounds, you can include 1 flexible carb, which means replacing 1 carb with around 100 flexible calories per day (1 carb serving is +/- 100 calories).
- If you weigh more than 200 pounds, 2 flexible carbs are okay. This means replacing up to 2 carbs with around 200 flexible calories (175–225 calorie range) per day.

Here is what 1 flexible carb looks like:

### ICE CREAM/FROZEN TREATS
- ¼–⅓ cup Ben & Jerry's
- ⅓–½ cup Breyers or Edy's
- ⅔ cup Halo Top
- ½ cup fruit-based sorbet
- ½ cup So Delicious coconut milk ice cream

### CHOCOLATE
- 2 tablespoons chocolate chips
- 5 Hershey's Kisses
- 1 pack M&M's, Fun Size
- 2 Ghirardelli chocolate squares, Intense Dark 92% Cacao or Sea Salt Caramel
- 1 ounce Lily's, dark chocolate or chocolate peanuts
- ¾ ounce HU Simple dark chocolate bar

### FRENCH FRIES
- ⅓ cup cooked from frozen
- McDonald's—children's menu size
- Wendy's—½ children's menu size
- ½ cup or ~2 ounces sweet potato fries, cooked from frozen

### POTATO CHIPS
- ⅔ cup or ¾ ounce traditional chips
- 1 single-serving bag or 1 ounce Popchips
- 1 ounce reduced-fat potato chips
- 1 ounce veggie straws, Sensible Portions

Flexible carbs are optional, not mandatory, and this list is just a set of examples—feel free to choose others. These foods tend to be higher in carbs and sugar yet lower in nutrients and fiber. That is what makes them flexible carbs.

Like a flexible carb, a flexible meal is an opportunity to satisfy a craving or make it easy to participate in social settings. One meal per week can be anything you desire: a pasta dish, pizza, a cheeseburger, anything fried, or a plate of nachos. Go wild. For some, two meals per week can still be appropriate if:

- You are making progress and would like the option of an additional flexible meal.
- You are feeling deprived or struggling to stick with the plan because of access to or preference for certain foods.
- Your starting weight is more than 200 pounds—this could mean your body can handle additional calories, carbs, and so on.
- You have no major medical issues like high cholesterol, high blood pressure, or high blood sugar. The additional faster-digesting carbs and saturated fat won't be as problematic.

Use your discretion and listen to hunger and fullness cues so that you're not eating past comfort. Knowing you have that weekly meal can also prevent overeating and support food freedom while you find your happiest weight.

## Using Alcohol As a Flexible Carb

Alcohol is not a carb, protein, or fat, but it is a source of calories. Considering that it is virtually empty calories, with little to no nutritional value, in Core Three it's called a flexible carb. A 100-calorie flexible carb is equivalent to:

- 1½ ounces (shot glass) of unflavored spirits or liquor
- 12 ounces (1 bottle) of "light" beer (darker beers are around 150–200 calories per 12 ounces)
- 5 ounces (half of a wine glass) of dry wine or champagne

Alcohol is not off the menu with the Core Three Plan, but it is important to drink responsibly and moderately. The American Heart Association considers moderation as one drink per day for women and two drinks per day for men. Males tend to have higher amounts of body water and of an enzyme called alcohol dehydrogenase, which breaks down alcohol. This helps men metabolize alcohol better than women, keeping their blood alcohol levels lower.

While you do have the option to replace a flexible carb with alcohol, keep in mind that it is a toxin and a depressant; it slows down your reflexes and movements. Alcohol also loosens inhibitions and interferes with sleep, which disrupts hormones that regulate appetite and hunger—specifically leptin and insulin. How often do you eat a pizza at 3:00 in the morning when not under the influence? While it's important not to think of that as a *bad* behavior, it is probably not helping you achieve your goals.

If you want to consider health, and potentially how you'll feel the next day, opt for beverages mixed with club soda and infused with lemon or lime. A 2017 study titled "Protective Effects of Lemon Juice on Alcohol-Induced Liver Injury in Mice" concluded that lemon juice can have protective benefits against liver injury related to chronic alcohol consumption. The researchers believe that it may be related to the antioxidant activity. You can also choose club soda (or soda water) with a splash of antioxidant-rich cranberry or pomegranate juice to make it taste sweeter. For many people, enjoying a cocktail, glass of wine, or vodka on the rocks can be a necessary part of socializing and living life. Think of alcohol as one of your treats that you can substitute for one to two carb servings and enjoy in moderation. This should also be said: If you struggle to limit your consumption, you may want to avoid alcohol intake entirely and seek help.

## Can I Have Caffeine?

If you're anything like me in the morning, it's "coffee first." Luckily, both coffee and tea can have a place in the Core Three. Helpfully, tea is a leading source of anti-oxidants. However, it is best to keep caffeine consumption under 400 milligrams per day. One 8-ounce cup of coffee has roughly 100 milligrams, and one espresso shot has about 65 milligrams. Of course, the average "cup" of coffee at a chain coffee shop can be closer to 12–16 ounces. One 8-ounce cup of black tea has just under 50

milligrams. Considering that caffeine is a stimulant, once the effects wear off, a crash will ensue and could lead to more intense hunger or cravings at the end of the day. Of course, the amount of caffeine in different beverages will vary, and individual caffeine tolerances depends upon the person.

Keep in mind that excessive caffeine can be dangerous for certain individuals. It is a stimulant that may exacerbate digestion issues such as acid reflux and nausea; can worsen mental health problems such as tension, nervousness, anxiety, and irritability; and can cause restlessness, palpitations, and even dizziness. Always exercise caution.

## Should I Supplement?

Supplements are meant to supplement foods in your diet, not replace them. Real foods reign supreme to supply your body with a necessary balance of nutrients. However, sometimes diet alone does not cut it. Here are a few supplements that might be warranted and why:

- **Multivitamin:** A multivitamin prevents nutritional deficiencies that can interfere with your health. Think of it like an insurance policy that can support healthy energy levels, whether your goal is to lose weight or not. While the Core Three is a nutrient-dense plan, a multivitamin can fill in any potential nutritional gaps.

- **Probiotics:** Probiotics are microorganisms—bacteria and yeast—that help balance the bacteria in your body. They are naturally found in your intestines but can easily be disrupted by stress, age, poor diet, medical issues, and medications. Dietary sources of probiotics include yogurt, kefir, kimchi, kombucha, and miso, but most of us don't consider these fermented foods dietary staples. A probiotic supplement with fifty billion colony-forming units (CFUs) of a variety of different strains can support better digestion and absorption of nutrients, along with a healthier metabolism.
- **Omega-3s (EPA/DHA):** Although you'll be working on eating more omega-3 fatty acids in your diet from salmon, tuna, grass-fed beef, and algae, it may come as a challenge. If you do not eat fatty fish regularly, a supplement is the next best option. Algae oil is an animal-free supplement that offers both EPA and DHA essential fatty acids.
- **B vitamins:** B vitamins help convert the food we eat into energy.
- **Magnesium:** Magnesium is critical for energy balance and can improve mood and digestion.
- **Vitamin D:** Vitamin D deficiency is a common issue and can impair the immune system, bone health, mood, and metabolism.
- **Other:** In Chapter 10, I cover more specific supplement recommendations based on special conditions.

Each person has different nutrient needs, but these supplements are all safe and beneficial for most healthy adults. Still, before you start any new supplements, it is important to consult with your doctor to ensure safety. Since the FDA does not regulate supplements, there might be discrepancies between the bottle label and what's inside the capsule. Fortunately, other companies have stepped in to provide quality testing and assurance. Look for a USP, NSF, or ConsumerLab seal for reassurance that the product is safe and reliable.

A successful eating plan should fit into your lifestyle—you shouldn't have to change your life to follow a plan. Combining what you *want* with what your body *needs* is ideal for finding your healthiest, happiest weight. It is also important to understand that personalization may continue as you make more progress over time. Continue to check in with how you're feeling, whether you're still achieving your goals, and what you could improve. In the next chapter, we will discuss additional ways to customize the plan based on special conditions.

# CHAPTER 10

# Adapting the Core Three for Special Conditions

Certain medical conditions can make it harder to find your happiest and healthiest weight—especially when you're dealing with hormonal disorders that affect insulin levels and metabolism. Disordered hormones can often lead to distorted views of your body and food. The good news is that your medical issues don't define your life or make you a flawed person who has to be "fixed." You might just have to work a little harder to accomplish your goals, lose weight, stay healthy, appreciate your body, and find food freedom. There are options for managing—and even overcoming—any health setbacks you may be experiencing. Just a few tweaks to the original Core Three formula can help you find success.

In this chapter, we will specifically explore how to adapt the plan for diabetes; PCOS; thyroid issues; the prenatal, postpartum, and postmenopausal phases; and eating disorders. You will learn about whether you should adjust specific macros, as well as certain foods to focus on and supplements that may help support your progress. I will also share a personal story about my own "special condition" and why I see it as a positive and not a negative. This chapter will offer tools to work with your body instead of against it.

**Special Note**

All these conditions should be managed with the help of trained healthcare professionals. Set up a time to talk with your doctor about your personal situation before adopting and/or adjusting the Core Three and taking any new supplements.

## Diabetes

There are four types of diabetes: type 1, type 2, prediabetes, and gestational diabetes. While none is directly caused by eating ice cream, cookies, or cake, all types denote high blood sugar levels, or hyperglycemia, and malfunctioning insulin. The good news is that the Core Three Healthy Eating Plan was designed to promote blood sugar stabilization.

### Type 1 Diabetes

Type 1 diabetes is an autoimmune disease that causes insulin deficiency and chronic high blood sugar levels (hyperglycemia). Insulin medication is required, regardless of how much or little you eat. The biggest misconception surrounding people with type 1 diabetes is that they must avoid sweets. People with type 1 diabetes can eat anything that people without diabetes can eat. They just need to adjust their insulin medication to compensate.

**ADAPTING THE CORE THREE**

Be prepared to lower, or adjust, your insulin medication as you change your diet.

- **Carbs:** If you're reducing carbohydrate intake, you will likely need to reduce insulin medication. In turn, this will encourage more fat-burning, making weight loss easier. Keep in mind that 1 Core Three carb serving equals around 20 grams of *net* carbs.

- **Proteins:** If you're eating significantly more protein, you may need additional insulin. Protein foods can be converted into glucose, although more slowly than carbohydrate foods.
- **Fats:** Anti-inflammatory fats should be the majority of your fat consumption.
- **Mindset:** Work on your relationship with food. NEDA's website explains that females with diabetes are "2.5 times more likely to develop eating disorders than those who do not have diabetes." An eating disorder can stem from years of feeling restricted and needing to control food intake beyond what is natural and normal.
- **Supplements:** Vitamin D deficiency can be a risk factor for developing type 1 diabetes and insulin malfunction. Eat more vitamin D–rich foods, such as dairy, oily fish, and eggs. Supplementing with 1,000–2,000 IU of vitamin D per day may be warranted if a deficiency is detected.

### Type 2 Diabetes

Type 2 diabetes is a metabolic disorder that leads to high blood glucose levels as a result of impaired insulin secretion and function. Healthy eating and exercise habits are vital and could potentially put you into remission without medication.

**ADAPTING THE CORE THREE PLAN**

A balanced, high-fiber diet is the key for balanced blood sugars.

- **Carbs:** Most healthy adults can include faster-digesting and lower-fiber carbs without any health implications. If you have diabetes, you don't have to cut out carbs, but it is more important to choose slower-digesting, higher-fiber carbs to stabilize your blood sugar and insulin levels.
- **Proteins:** People with diabetes often have higher inflammation levels, so limit LDL cholesterol-spiking saturated fats (that's the "lousy" cholesterol I talked about in Chapter 6). Aim for at least 6–9 ounces of oily, fatty fish per week, and incorporate some plant proteins. Use the Plant-Based Proteins chart in Chapter 5 to see how they convert into carb exchanges, so that you can still keep blood sugar levels stable.
- **Fats:** Eating more oily, fatty fish or taking an omega-3 (EPA/DHA) supplement will help fight low-grade systemic inflammation that is often present in people with diabetes. Otherwise, choose more MUFAs like extra-virgin olive oil and avocado from the Mono- and Polyunsaturated Fats chart in Chapter 6.
- **Additional foods:** Load up on non-starchy vegetables. Limit alcohol and caffeine, which can interfere with blood sugar levels.
- **Exercise:** Aim for at least 90 minutes of insulin-sensitizing strength training exercises per week as part of your weekly 3 hours.

- **Specific supplements to consider:**
  - **Chromium picolinate:** Chromium picolinate is a mineral that plays a major role in blood glucose control and reducing insulin resistance. This essential nutrient is found in various foods, including fruits, veggies, whole grains, and meats. While it may seem simple to consume enough from your diet, according to a scientific review called "The Role of Chromium in Insulin Resistance," published in the medical journal *Diabetes Education*, "dietary chromium is poorly absorbed." The review also explains that "chromium levels decrease with age," and therefore a daily supplement "containing 200–1,000 mcg chromium as chromium picolinate" is the best way to ensure optimal absorption.
  - **Curcumin/turmeric:** There is strong evidence that curcumin (the active compound in turmeric) can lower blood glucose levels and fight insulin resistance. You may notice benefits if you take 500 milligrams of curcumin per day for at least 4 weeks.
  - **Resveratrol:** Resveratrol, which has antioxidant properties, can improve glycemic control and decrease insulin resistance. Recommended intake is around 250–500 milligrams per day.

Always consult with your doctor before taking any new supplements to ensure there are no contraindications.

### Prediabetes

Prediabetes is often diagnosed when your blood sugar levels start to rise but are not quite high enough to qualify as type 2 diabetes. Your eating habits should mimic those of someone with type 2 diabetes; therefore, you can use the same guidelines.

### Gestational Diabetes

Gestational diabetes is diagnosed during pregnancy through an oral glucose tolerance test. It often resolves itself after delivery. Of course, weight loss during pregnancy is not advised and can be dangerous. Eat a *minimum* of three servings of each food group and wait until after pregnancy to start on this plan.

## What Is PCOS?

PCOS is a prevalent female condition that is characterized as a hormonal imbalance with high levels of androgens, also known as "male hormones," and potentially underlying insulin resistance. Symptoms include irregular periods, acne, abnormal hair growth, and difficulty losing body fat, especially around the midsection. For that reason, it is no surprise that women with PCOS often struggle with poor body image and distorted eating.

Although PCOS is complex and symptoms can vary from person to person, it is manageable. Most of my PCOS clients are often advised to "lose weight" or "eliminate carbs" to treat any unwanted symptoms and fight insulin resistance. However, the most effective, healthiest treatment involves a balanced diet, regular exercise, and targeted supplements.

### Adapting the Core Three

Stabilizing blood sugars and reducing inflammation through your diet is key.

- **Carbs:** Don't cut out carbs entirely. Carbs are the primary source of soluble fiber that can boost metabolism and lead to a healthier gut. Carbs also provide anti-inflammatory antioxidants and an assortment of other nutrients, such as chromium, B vitamins, vitamin C, magnesium, and iron, all of which are key for energy, metabolism, and hormonal balance. Stick with slower-digesting carbs and consider reducing 1 serving of carbohydrates per day only if you're not noticing any progress. For example, if you're hovering around 4–5 carbohydrates per day, then reduce to 3 or 4.
  - **Should you go gluten-free?** Gluten is a protein found in wheat, barley, and rye, so any product that contains one of these grains will contain gluten. There is no conclusive evidence to support

gluten-free eating to treat PCOS symptoms. Yet some women find relief and notice improvements in different areas, including clearer skin and accelerated weight loss. Anecdotally, limiting gluten might be something to consider, but only if you can do so safely and easily. Going gluten-free can be hard to sustain and make it more difficult to obtain the recommended 25-plus grams of fiber per day. If you do want to attempt a gluten-free diet, make sure it is a realistic commitment and that it does not leave you feeling more stressed around mealtimes. You can also consider replacing gluten with nongluten foods for 3–4 weeks and then slowly add it back in to determine if your body has a true reaction. After the 4 weeks are up, I suggest starting with a half slice of whole-wheat bread on day one, then a whole slice of bread on day two, and then two slices of bread on day three. If you don't notice any reactions 48 hours after day three, then you likely tolerate gluten. If you do notice a reaction, then you can continue to look for replacements. Most gluten-free foods will have it written on the label. Look for gluten-free products that have at least 2–3 grams of fiber per serving.

- **Protein:** Aim for at least 6–9 ounces of omega-3 fatty acids to fight inflammation. Include plant proteins as often as possible. Consider choosing more organic and grass-fed animal foods.

- **Should you limit dairy?** It is not necessary to limit cow's milk, but, as with gluten, certain individuals with PCOS report an increase in symptoms after eating dairy. This is due to a common farming practice that involves injecting cows with a growth hormone to increase milk supply. While the FDA maintains that dairy is perfectly safe for human consumption, other research shows it could be cause for concern only in susceptible populations—like those with hormonal imbalances and underlying insulin resistance. The issue with ditching dairy is that yogurt is a leading source of probiotics, which are important for hormone function, and vitamin D, which helps promotes insulin and glucose regulation. Some research shows dairy can have an anti-inflammatory effect when consumed in moderation. Additional studies include full-fat dairy as an important food group for fertility. That said, going dairy-free or reducing dairy might help alleviate specific symptoms for certain individuals, especially if you have a sensitivity to dairy proteins or milk sugar (lactose). There are several dairy-free yogurt and milk options listed in the Core Three food tables in Chapters 4–7 to make it easier to find substitutes if you want to experiment. Keep in mind that avoiding dairy like yogurt, milk, and cheese can be hard to sustain, so choose this route only if you truly suspect dairy doesn't agree with you. The best approach is to do a simple elimination diet, where you substitute it out for just 3–4 weeks and then slowly reintroduce to see if you notice any changes in symptoms, ovulation, acne, energy, or weight. You can start with 1 ounce of cheese, and then 2 ounces of cheese the next day, and then 3 ounces of cheese on the third day. Forty-eight hours after the third day, if you experience additional symptoms, continue to replace cow's milk dairy with plant-based versions.

- **Fats:** Stick with mostly anti-inflammatory fats.
  - **Try incorporating pumpkin seeds.** These are a powerhouse of nutrients that are effective in fighting PCOS symptoms. They contain beta-sitosterol, which interferes with the enzyme that converts testosterone to dihydrotestosterone (DHT). DHT is a hormone that can shrink hair follicles, leading to hormonal hair loss, commonly seen in PCOS. Not everyone with PCOS notices hair loss—it depends on your sensitivity to DHT. It is also possible to have normal levels of testosterone in blood work but experience DHT-related hair loss anyway. Pumpkin seeds are also an important anti-inflammatory fat that provides a plethora of other nutrients, such as zinc, magnesium, iron, antioxidants, and fiber. All these nutrients work together to promote healthier hair, stabilize blood sugar levels and weight, and help regulate menstrual cycles. If you're not a pumpkin seed enthusiast, taking a pumpkin seed oil supplement can offer a more concentrated dose of DHT-blocking beta-sitosterol. Look for a supplement with about 1,000 milligrams; you can take it in capsule or liquid form. Keep in mind that hair growth restoration may not be noticeable for about 6 months, so you have to be patient as the regrowth cycle takes time.

- **Exercise:** Aim for at least 90 minutes of resistance training exercise per week as part of the recommended 3 hours total. Building lean muscle can help improve insulin sensitivity and reregulate hormones. Overexercising may further stress out your body and complicate hormonal harmony, so don't overdo it.

- **Supplements:** Add in specific supplements that target insulin resistance:

  - **Inositol:** Inositol is a vitamin-like substance that your body naturally produces. It can come in a variety of forms; however, a 2014 study published in the *European Review for Medical and Pharmacological Sciences* determined that patients who received myo-inositol and/or D-chiro-inositol administration showed improved insulin sensitivity. A ratio of forty to one (myo-inositol to D-chiro-inositol) appears to be the optimal dose for insulin resistance and therefore weight management.

  - **Green tea extract:** Green tea is an incredible source of anti-inflammatory antioxidants that can also help rebalance hormones. A 2017 clinical trial published in the *Journal of Education and Health Promotion* discovered that the consumption of 500 milligrams of green tea extract twice daily for 12 weeks led to weight loss, decreased fasting insulin levels, and lower levels of free testosterone in overweight women with PCOS.

  - **Resveratrol:** Resveratrol is a powerful polyphenol found naturally in the skins of red grapes, red wine, peanuts, and blueberries. It shows promise for fighting against insulin resistance and inflammation at therapeutic doses of 500–1,000 milligrams per day.

  - **Berberine:** Berberine is a naturally occurring organic compound derived from various plant sources. An abundance of research suggests that berberine is an effective insulin sensitizer that has similar action on the body to metformin, but without the side effects. It can help promote fat-burning, especially around the tummy area. Recommended doses are 500–1,500 milligrams per day; however, you should get your doctor's okay before trying it.

- **Work on body image.** Losing weight can be difficult when you have PCOS. Have self-compassion and be gentle and patient with yourself.

Living with PCOS can be difficult, but I firmly believe that when you focus only on the issues, the issues get bigger. When you shift your focus to solutions, the solutions become bigger. With proper care and management of symptoms, you can have a fulfilling, healthy, and happy future. Trust me, I know.

### Let's Get Personal

In 2016 after tying the knot with my husband, I finally untied the knot with a much longer relationship: birth control pills. My plan was to stop the pill so we could start a family. Not long after that, I quickly discovered that when it comes to fertility, there is no such thing as planning. An issue had been lurking inside my body, masked by synthetic hormones, for over a decade. It was like my OB-GYN slapped me across the face when she sat me down and said, "You have PCOS." Of course, no one with PCOS should feel flawed, but when you hear the news for the first time, it can be incredibly difficult to process.

Not long after I received the diagnosis, the symptoms abruptly started. My hair was shedding, my skin was breaking out, and my emotions were all over the place. Most medications that can instantly treat these symptoms are dangerous for a woman who's trying to conceive, as they can affect fetal development. Here I was, dealing with all these issues, and to add insult to injury, I was suffering through one failed ovulation cycle after another.

I knew I had to take more action. I scoured the Internet and all my professional resources for books, studies, experts, and everything in between. Sure, as a dietitian, I had a basic understanding of how to treat PCOS. Yet, when you're the one being diagnosed, there is a deeper level of determination to find answers and solution. Probably the best thing that came from this whole experience was that I now understand more than ever how my clients feel. The major revelation was that

there is an overwhelming number of theories, books, and experts who are making millions on bold PCOS promises that are not based on good science. The truth is, everyone is different, and the best treatment option is the one that's best tailored to fit your specific case. Some women can successfully send their PCOS symptoms into remission through a combination of lifestyle changes, including diet and exercise. I have witnessed it with my clients! Others find that it's not so simple and may need to incorporate medications like a birth control pill, spironolactone, and metformin, all of which can tackle the hormonal imbalance and mitigate issues like acne, hair loss, and potentially weight changes. The most realistic expectation, and one that you should absolutely believe, is that there is something you can do about it. If your main concern is fertility, I promise you that there is hope.

Fortunately, I have been able to manage my symptoms through a balanced diet, moderate exercise, and other lifestyle changes. At some point, I may get back on the birth control pill for additional assistance if I need to. That's my prerogative—and it should be yours too. Thanks to reproductive technology, I was also able to successfully have children—twin boys—and have made my peace with PCOS. I will never forget what my fertility endocrinologist said to me when I nervously met with him for an initial consultation: "Of all the fertility issues you can have, PCOS is by far the easiest to work with." Work with your PCOS, not against it. It does not have to define your life.

## Thyroid Issues

"Do you think it's my thyroid?" This is one of the most common questions I am asked when working with women who are struggling to lose weight. In some cases, the answer is yes! Your thyroid controls metabolism, influencing how much energy your body requires.

There are four predominant thyroid conditions: hypothyroidism, Hashimoto's disease, hyperthyroidism, and Graves' disease. All affect metabolism, but they should be treated a little differently.

### Hypothyroidism
One of the more commonly diagnosed thyroid conditions, hypothyroidism means you have an underactive thyroid.

#### ADAPTING THE CORE THREE
Be prepared to make some tweaks along the way.

- **Carbs:** Choose slower-digesting carbs, as blood sugar imbalance can contribute to thyroid hormone imbalance. One influences the other. Be prepared to take out 1 carb serving if you don't notice progress. Especially while you're trying to up your T3 and T4

hormones through medication, your metabolism may be a little late to the party.
- **Proteins:** Consume fatty fish and, if possible, choose wild over farm-raised to minimize contaminants that can further disrupt the endocrine system. Otherwise, a variety of animal and plant proteins is ideal for maximum absorption of nutrients that support thyroid function, such as B vitamins, iron, iodine, and zinc.
- **Fats:** Aside from anti-inflammatory fats, consuming coconut oil in moderation may be beneficial. Coconut oil contains medium-chain triglycerides that have a positive effect on fullness and energy and can increase metabolism.
- **Nutrients:** Supplements can help correct deficiencies, but always consult with your doctor before taking anything new. Core nutrients to pay attention to for hypothyroidism include:
  - **Iodine:** This vital nutrient is used to make thyroid hormones and is mostly found in seafood like fish, as well as sea vegetables, dairy, and iodized salt. Insufficient iodine intake can be a main contributor to thyroid conditions and a potentially slowed metabolism.
  - **Selenium:** Selenium is a necessary component of enzymes that directly support thyroid function. It is found mostly in nuts, seeds,

and whole grains, but the best source of selenium is Brazil nuts. Consuming just one Brazil nut per day supplies all the selenium you need.

- **Zinc:** This mineral is required for thyroid hormone production and for balancing out TSH, T3, and T4. Oysters are the richest source of zinc, followed by red meat, poultry, seafood, beans, nuts, whole grains, and dairy products.
- **Iron:** Iron deficiency can impair thyroid function, and sufficient iron levels are important for T4 to T3 conversion. Iron-dense foods include lean meat, seafood, poultry, iron-fortified cereals, beans,

## Finding Relief for Constipation

A sluggish thyroid can also lead to a sluggish digestive tract and constipation. This can make you feel heavier and uncomfortable. When it comes to constipation, the first line of defense is:

- A high-fiber diet (more than 25 grams per day)
- Plenty of water (2–3 liters daily)
- Moderate exercise (around 3 hours per week)

All of these are emphasized with the Core Three Healthy Eating Plan. Here are a few additional natural constipation remedies for when you need an extra bowel movement boost:

- **Chia and flax seeds:** Just 1–2 tablespoons per day can help push waste through your intestines. Both are key sources of soluble fiber that forms a gel after digestion for a better-formed bowel movement.
- **Magnesium citrate:** Magnesium is a naturally occurring mineral that plays a vital role in the body. It is important for energy, muscles, and nerve function. It is also used to treat constipation, as it pulls water into the intestines, encouraging passage of waste. Follow the instructions on the label and consult with a gastroenterologist first to rule out any other medical issues that may warrant closer attention. Magnesium-rich foods include spinach, avocado, almonds, and pumpkin seeds.
- **Vitamin C:** Like magnesium, this powerful, immune-supporting antioxidant can attract water into the intestines to fight constipation. Start with 1,000 milligrams per day and do not exceed the upper limit (2,000 milligrams per day) unless under medical supervision. Vitamin C can also be found in foods like citrus fruits, tomatoes, red peppers, strawberries, broccoli, and spinach.

lentils, spinach, peas, nuts, and some dried fruits.

- **Vitamin B1 (thiamine):** Eating more thiamine-rich foods can fight fatigue, which is a common hypothyroidism symptom. Thiamine is predominantly found in sunflower seeds, navy beans, oats, asparagus, sweet potatoes, lentils, and lima beans.

## Hashimoto's Thyroiditis

Hashimoto's is an autoimmune condition that involves your immune system attacking your thyroid gland.

### ADAPTING THE CORE THREE

Hashimoto's symptoms are similar to those of hypothyroidism and include poor energy and difficulty losing weight. If you're not making progress using the original Core Three formula, you can address it in the following ways:

- **Carbs:** Subtract 1 carbohydrate serving, unless you're already at 3 carbs per day. You can also subtract 1 protein and 1 fat per day, if you're portioning those out as well. Wait 3 weeks, see how you feel, and then repeat if necessary.
- **Proteins:** A variety of proteins from plant and animal sources is ideal for nutrient balance. Consuming at least 6–9 ounces of fatty, oily fish for inflammation-fighting essential

omega-3s is also important. While most healthy adults do not need to stress over wild versus farmed-raised seafood, farmed fish tend to have higher levels of contaminants such as polychlorinated biphenyls (PCBs). PCBs are a type of chemical that can be considered toxic in large quantities and disrupt your endocrine system and hormonal harmony. The US Environmental Protection Agency maintains that farmed fish tend to have higher levels of contaminants compared with wild fish, which can be a concern in certain populations. In that case, opt for wild salmon and other fish whenever possible. Canned Pacific sockeye salmon is low in PCBs, shelf-stable, and less expensive than fresh fish. (In Chapter 14, you'll find a Simple Salmon Croquettes recipe that uses canned salmon and a few other ingredients.) If you are not an avid fish eater for one reason or another, you can take an omega-3 supplement. Algae (algal) oil supplements are vegan and virtually PCB-free and contain an effective balance of EPA and DHA fatty acids. Ideally, aim for around 250–500 milligrams of EPA and DHA combined per day. Check supplement labels to confirm.

- **Fats:** Eat a variety of anti-inflammatory fats and try to incorporate coconut oil on occasion as well. Replace higher-omega-6 oils, such as corn, soybean, sunflower, safflower, and cottonseed, with more anti-inflammatory oils like extra-virgin olive oil or avocado oil.

- **Nutrients:** Before starting any supplements, it's important to consult with your endocrinologist or whoever is treating your thyroid conditions. Getting tested for possible deficiencies is the first step to determine if supplements may be warranted. Additional core nutrients for Hashimoto's are as follows:
  - **Vitamin D:** There is a link between D deficiency and Hashimoto's; however, it is unclear which comes first. Regardless, if you are vitamin D deficient, supplementation is important. Most blood tests ring the alarm only if your D levels fall under 30 ng/ml, but many integrative nutrition experts prefer higher than 50 ng/ml. Vitamin D–rich foods include cod liver oil, salmon, swordfish, tuna, dairy, egg yolks, and fortified juices/cereals.
  - **Magnesium:** A magnesium deficiency may increase the risk of developing autoimmune Hashimoto's and is associated with elevated thyroid antibody levels. Correcting your levels can improve symptoms, especially constipation and mood changes.

## Hyperthyroidism

Hyperthyroidism is what it sounds like—a hyperactive thyroid. It goes into rapid fire, and this butterfly-shaped organ overproduces T3 and T4 hormones, while TSH remains below normal range.

### ADAPTING THE CORE THREE

As with hypothyroidism, vitamin D, selenium, magnesium, and B vitamins can help with thyroid function. However, limiting iodine intake and increasing goitrogenic foods can help stabilize thyroid hormones. It may also be particularly helpful to limit caffeine.

## Graves' Disease

Graves' disease is the autoimmune variant of hyperthyroidism. As in Hashimoto's, the body attacks its own cells, which leads to an overproduction of T3 and T4 hormones.

### ADAPTING THE CORE THREE

- **Carbs, proteins, and fats:** Follow the guidelines for hyperthyroidism, with a special attention to anti-inflammatory fats like fish oils, avocado, and extra-virgin olive oil.
- **Additional ideas:** Ruling out food sensitivities, focusing on gut health, and experimenting with a gluten- and soy-free diet may also help treat Graves' disease symptoms.

## Additional Thyroid Recommendations

Most thyroid conditions are managed through medications. However, diet can still help manage lingering symptoms. The Core Three Plan will be particularly helpful to improve energy, fight constipation, and assist with weight management or weight loss. The following are some additional ideas that can help manage thyroid conditions:

### GOITROGENIC FOODS

Goitrogenic foods are a range of foods that can interfere with thyroidal iodine uptake and impair thyroid peroxidase activity, thus impeding thyroid hormone regulation. While most dietary goitrogens have minimal impact unless consumed raw or in large quantities, it is important to familiarize yourself with what these are:

- Cruciferous vegetables: cabbage, kale, cauliflower, broccoli, turnips, rapeseed
- Cassava, lima beans, sweet potato, sorghum
- Flavonoids found in soy, millet, red wine, green tea, spinach, legumes

Cooking destroys up to 90 percent of the goitrogenic properties in these foods, so be sure to roast, steam, sauté, or bake when possible.

### LEARN ABOUT LECTIN FOODS

Lectins are a naturally occurring protein found in most plants—they are unavoidable. Lectins are highest in legumes, grains, and nightshade vegetables like tomatoes, potatoes, eggplant, peppers, and seed spices. A lower-lectin diet may be helpful for some autoimmune disorders, but studies are mixed. Cooking destroys most of the potentially harmful effects of lectins, such as interfering with nutrient absorption, causing damage to the digestive tract, and increasing inflammation. Certain lectin-containing foods, such as beans, can be poisonous if not cooked or if undercooked. However, for those with sensitive conditions, including poor digestion, arthritis, and autoimmune conditions like Hashimoto's and Graves' disease, limiting lectin foods may help manage symptoms.

### GO WITH YOUR GUT

A healthy digestive system that allows for proper absorption and metabolism is imperative, especially for the thyroid. Tips for improving gut health include:

- Eat 25–35 grams of fiber per day.
- Eat more prebiotic-rich foods, like bananas, garlic, onions, and leeks.
- Eat more fermented, probiotic-rich foods, like yogurt with live and active cultures, kefir, kombucha, and sauerkraut.
- Take a daily probiotic supplement with at least 50 billion CFUs and a variety of strains.
- Add in L-glutamine through supplementation; it is an amino acid that

can support gut wall strength to prevent leaky gut syndrome, or intestinal permeability.

**GIVE UP ON GLUTEN?**

The final dietary adjustment that may help certain individuals is a low-gluten or gluten-free diet. While it is not advised to completely avoid any food if you are working on your overall relationship with food, some discover symptom cessation as a result of cutting out gluten. Studies show that gluten can lead to the production of zonulin, a protein that modulates the integrity of cell walls in the digestive tract. When overproduced, this recently discovered modulator can contribute to intestinal damage, which allows passage of molecules through the gut barrier, increasing immune response and further exacerbating autoimmune conditions like Hashimoto's. If you suspect a sensitivity to gluten, eliminate gluten-containing foods for only a short period of time (3–4 weeks) before determining whether you're better off with or without it. If you don't notice any changes, slowly reintroduce it.

## Postpartum Planning

When you first make that major, life-changing decision to start a family, you want to make sure you do whatever you can to ensure it's smooth sailing. Going on a diet, cutting down on specific foods,

and overexercising can be stressful on your body and impact fertility. Prenatally, you can still follow the basic guidelines of the Core Three, including a minimum of each group. However, it is not the best time to fixate on weight loss.

If you're past the point of pregnancy and are blessed with a newborn baby, you might be eager to get your prepregnancy body back. But immediately bouncing back to your prebaby body is not necessary or realistic. If you're breastfeeding, your body may be even more resistant to returning to its prepregnancy state. Although it might be hard to accept your body the way it is, try to practice self-compassion. You have gone through a lot! The pressure is powerful, but it is best to take it slow with weight loss for the following reasons:

- **It can decrease your milk supply.** Producing milk requires sufficient calories and nutrients. Restricting foods can lead to decreased milk supply, which is a major stressor, especially when you have a wailing hangry baby in your arms.
- **Your skin can sag.** Even if you lose all the pounds you gained during pregnancy, your skin might not appreciate the shortcut. Quick weight loss can lead to increased skin sagging. Slow and steady wins the race, especially when it comes to preserving skin elasticity.
- **It can affect your mood and emotions.** Restricting what you eat

while trying to juggle being a new mom with other life responsibilities is just as overwhelming as it sounds. Even following a healthy weight loss plan requires a degree of focus, energy, and patience—but at this point, you need to devote most of those things to your newborn. Further, you could be missing out on key nutrients like vitamin D, omega-3s, and magnesium that help with mood and emotional stability. The first few months with your little one will pretty much demand all that and more. What's most important is that you're feeling mentally and physically healthy, whether or not your weight is where you want it to be.

## Adapting the Core Three

If you are nursing, then you should eat as if you were pregnant. In some cases, women can actually burn more calories while breastfeeding than during pregnancy. If you are not breastfeeding, your body still needs replenishment of nutrients that can be lost throughout pregnancy and delivery. For that reason, you can still follow the following guidelines.

- **Carbs, proteins, and fats:** If your baby is starting to wean off breast-milk and eating more solids, then you can likely start to gradually cut back on servings of carbohydrates. I recommend starting slow by taking out 1 daily carb and then waiting at least 3 weeks before determining how your body is responding. Continue choosing high-fiber carbs, lean proteins, and anti-inflammatory fats for optimal energy, recovery, and healing. If you're starting to notice positive changes, great, but if not, you can take out one additional serving from another category, such as proteins or fats. Do not go below the original Core Three Healthy Eating Plan recommendations.

- **Milk supply:** If you notice your milk supply is starting to dry up, you will need to add back in at least one portion of each category if you wish to continue breastfeeding.

- **Exercise:** You can increase exercise gradually after you receive clearance to do so from your doctor, to reach the weekly 3 hours—but only if you have the time and energy. As a new mom, you're likely getting more than enough activity, especially if you're nursing. Exercising when you're sleep-deprived is counterproductive—your body won't respond well to movement without adequate rest. Pushing yourself too much in the form of exercise, or restrictive eating, can significantly impact recovery and well-being.

- **Hydration:** Hydration is so important when you're lactating. Aim for the high end of 2–3 liters per day and continue taking a prenatal vitamin until you're completely done breastfeeding.

After that you can switch to a regular multivitamin, as your body likely does not need the extra nutrients in a prenatal, such as folic acid or iron.

## Postmenopausal

Menopause refers to the point when a woman stops menstruation, or no longer has a true period. At this stage, ovaries stop producing eggs and the female hormones, estrogen and progesterone, decline. This unavoidable juncture in life can leave you feeling pretty crappy. What's worse is that you're made to think it's all just a "normal" part of aging and you should just accept it. Many younger women believe they won't worry as much about how they look or feel when they're older. But very few, if any, women, middle-aged or older, ever say that. Feeling confident about your appearance can affect your quality of life, and you deserve to feel your best, regardless of what's going on inside your body. Your chronological age does not have to mimic your biological age, or how old you feel.

Weight loss can be more difficult for postmenopausal women due to the fluctuation or plummeting of female hormones, muscle loss, and lifestyle changes. But taking care of yourself is not less important when you're fifty, sixty, seventy, or even eighty—it's actually more important than ever! Quality of life will drastically improve with proper self-care. Combining a healthy

eating plan, moderate exercise, adequate sleep, and stress management can help you feel more youthful, regardless of your birth year.

**Adapting the Core Three**
You might find that following the standard Core Three Healthy Eating Plan still works for you, but if it doesn't, you can make some adjustments.

- **Carbs:** If you're eating more than 3 carbs a day, cut down 1 carb—for example, if you're instructed to eat 4 carbs per day, reduce to 3 per day. Choose lower-glycemic carbs with higher fiber content that will promote stable blood sugar and insulin levels. Insulin resistance risk increases with age.
- **Proteins:** Add in one additional serving of protein. Animal foods are also the best source of collagen, which can improve skin elasticity, strengthen connective tissues, and alleviate join pain. A collagen supplement with hydrolyzed collagen peptides is effectively absorbed, can help mitigate normal wear and tear, and can improve gut lining as well. Because collagen can significantly decline with aging, a supplement can provide a subtle boost to your fragile connective tissue and skin.
- **Fats:** Fats, along with proper hydration, are particularly beneficial for health of skin, hair, and nails, so

be sure you are eating a variety of anti-inflammatory fats and coconut oil in moderation.

- **Exercise:** Strength training is a must for metabolism and healthy bones. Aim for at least 2 hours (of the 3 recommended hours) per week.

## Disordered Eating and Eating Disorders

If you have a history of an eating disorder or a suspected eating disorder, any part of this plan can be triggering. In fact, any program that provides instructions on how much to eat can instill irrational fears. If you're still in the thick of recovering from an eating disorder, this plan is not advised unless under medical supervision.

The Core Three is about choosing higher-fiber carbs, lean proteins, and anti-inflammatory fats, but when you have a special condition, it is even more beneficial to opt for these specific types of macronutrients. Continue to work on your relationship with food and other lifestyle habits like moderate exercise, adequate sleep, and stress management. Your body is like an orchestra: When everything is in the right place at the right time, you will find that harmony and healthy weight loss will be much easier.

**CHAPTER 11**

# Sustaining Your Success

Now that you have a healthy and personalized eating plan, how are you going to set yourself up to sustain these results? Executing behaviors and turning them into long-term habits are the final steps to solidifying your success. The key is to focus on what is helping you achieve your goals and acknowledge certain actions that are sabotaging your efforts. Manifest what you wish to achieve by showing up for yourself, putting in the effort, and staying positive. Whether you wish to lose weight, improve your relationship with food and your body, or just feel healthier, you must have an action plan and believe it is possible. Imagine the type of life that you desire—and deserve—to live. Now go and live it.

In this chapter, I'll teach you the best ways to set yourself up for success. This includes how to make permanent behavior changes and track your progress to help you stay mindful and motivated, because when you rely solely on the scale to determine success, it can do more harm than good. I'll discuss why food journaling is so important in helping to keep you accountable, especially in the beginning. You'll also learn how to find your healthiest, happiest weight and why slow weight loss prevails. Finally, we will talk about how to make lasting behavioral changes for long-term success.

## Tracking Your Progress

When it comes to improvements with your body, you will often feel them before you see them. Look out for the following differences:

- Improved energy
- Better digestion (less acid reflux, constipation, and stomach bloating)
- More restful sleep
- Enhanced concentration and creativity
- Upbeat and more stable mood
- Increased calm and peace around food
- Fewer feelings of deprivation or disorder
- Improvements in blood work (cholesterol, triglycerides, liver enzymes, blood sugars)

These changes require a degree of mindfulness and paying attention to your body. Of course, your friends and family won't be as quick to pay you compliments about your improved digestion or cholesterol levels. But that doesn't mean they're not just as, if not more, valuable measures of health than going down a size in clothes.

## Stepping on the Scale

Most people rely on frequent weigh-ins to track weight loss progress. While regular scale usage can be helpful to stay on track, it can also be discouraging and not all that accurate. For that reason, the Core Three Plan only recommends *stepping on a scale no more than once a week, or about three times per month (skipping the week that you're about to get your period, if you have a menstrual cycle). It is also best to weigh in the morning before you have eaten anything and after you go to the bathroom.* Weighing in on a Wednesday-to-Friday cycle can also help you obtain a more accurate read, according to a study published in the *Obesity Facts: The European Journal of Obesity,* titled "Weight Rhythms: Weight Increases during Weekends and Decreases during Weekdays." That's because weekend eating is often different from weekday eating. Meals are spaced differently and can be heavier in carbs or sodium—all of which can affect water weight and, thus, the scale. So, instead of following a 7-day weekly weigh-in schedule, extend it another few days.

### SORTING OUT THE SCALE

Aside from time of day and day of week, there are other reasons why scales are so problematic.

- **Fluid shifts:** The majority of your total body weight (about 60 percent) is water, and only a small percentage is pure body fat. Now consider how much your water weight can fluctuate throughout the month, week, and even day as a result of eating, sweating, or going to the bathroom.
- **Muscle changes:** You might not see muscle mass changes right away, but

over time they can show up on the scale. If you have been doing more resistance training, the scale may go up instead of down. Don't mistake that for a lack of progress. It simply means the scale might not reflect real body fat changes so accurately.

- **Hormonal fluctuations:** Another factor to consider is hormones, particularly estrogen and progesterone. They can influence so many functions in your body, especially your weight. The scale can fluctuate 2–3 pounds, if not more, in the days leading up to a new menstrual cycle. A 2015 study in the *International Journal of Women's Health* concluded that approximately 92 percent of women report bloat and edema in the second part of their cycle, aka the luteal phase. For that reason, I highly suggest avoiding the scale altogether for the entire week before and a few days after your period presents itself.

- **Bowel movement regularity:** If you struggle with constipation, you'll see that reflected on the scale. An individual can hold up to 4 pounds of fecal matter when constipated. (See Chapter 10 for constipation-relieving tips.)

All these circumstances can affect what digits are blinking back at you under your feet. You cannot always take that number at face value—you may not see any movement for a couple of weeks, and then may notice you've lost a few pounds all at once.

If you decide to use the scale, make sure it is helping and not harming your progress.

### Obsessed with the Scale? Ditch It Altogether

If you find yourself becoming obsessive with or dependent on the scale, weighing in multiple times per day, it is likely affecting your mood and happiness. If you automatically get discouraged by the number you see or you allow yourself to eat certain foods only when that number is down, it's time to pack it up, put it away, and come back to it later. Finding scale-free successes is key to prevent burnout and reinforce positive behaviors. Know that you deserve to be happy with your body despite what the scale says.

### Using Body Composition Analysis

As mentioned in Chapter 1, measuring your body fat, muscle, and water weight is more productive than just total pounds. If you know these individual measurements, you can easily detect changes in muscle mass and body fat to ensure you're heading in the intended direction. Yet it is still a number, and there can still be discrepancies and variables at play. As with the scale, many factors can affect the accuracy of body fat analysis. Proceed with caution if you tend to get easily discouraged by numbers or rely on them for validation. We'll discuss body composition more later in this chapter.

## How to Find Your Happiest, Healthiest Weight

Your "happy weight" is a weight, size, or body composition at which you feel comfortable and confident without feeling tied to chronic exercise or extreme food deprivation. If you're not sure what your happy weight is, the following questions can help provide more insight:

- **What is your age, height, and sex?** These objective measures can help piece together what is feasible. The taller you are, the more mass your body may carry. A 5-foot person who was assigned female at birth has a much different body size than a 6-foot person who was assigned male at birth. To determine a healthy weight range, I start with the Hamwi "Ideal Weight" Formula.
  - For females: Start with 100 pounds for the first 5 feet of height and add in 5 pounds for each additional inch. For example, if you're 5-foot-4, your ideal weight would calculate at 120 pounds. Add and subtract 10 percent for a range. This translates to 108–132 pounds. This range allows for variances in muscle mass, body frame size, and age. This does not mean if you're 5-foot-4, and weigh over 132 pounds you are automatically unhealthy. It just means that your body might not be designed, or genetically capable, of going down in that range.
  - For males: Start with 106 pounds per 5 feet and add in 6 pounds for each additional inch of height. If you're a 6-foot male, this translates to 178 pounds plus or minus 10 percent, or 160–196 pounds. Of course, this is still just a number and only a total poundage. Use this range as a starting point, but it might need to be tweaked based on the following questions.
- **What was your lowest adult weight (age eighteen and older), and has your lifestyle changed?** If your goal weight is a size you saw only in your teenage years, you may want to reconsider. Comparing your adult body to your sixteen-year-old self is not realistic. Your body may not be fully developed until you are well over age eighteen. There may be a good reason you never reached that size as an adult—your body is telling you it's not healthy. Even if you have seen that number on the scale, what were the circumstances? Was it after a bad bout of food poisoning? Were you living in the city and walking everywhere? Was this pre-family when you only had to worry about yourself? Was it on your wedding day, when you had a gown to squeeze into that hundreds of guests were eager to see, with a professional

photographer waiting to permanently capture it? If you weighed that amount only because of fleeting circumstances, it may not be your healthiest size.

- **What is your highest adult weight?** If this is your highest adult weight, then healthy weight loss is possible. However, if you are well below your highest, perhaps there is not much more weight you can safely lose. As you lose weight, your metabolism can slow (this is natural and normal), making it extra difficult to keep losing weight in a healthy, safe manner. Pushing it too far past where you are now can slow your metabolism down even more and cause rebound weight gain.

- **What is your body composition?** Total pounds don't account for body fat versus muscle mass. Instead of fixating on a total number of pounds, aim for a healthier body fat percentage, which is roughly 18–30 percent for females and 10–20 percent for males. After all, who cares if you gained a few pounds on the scale if it was mostly muscle?

## Why Is Slow Weight Loss Important?

When it comes to weight loss, slow and steady wins the race. Healthy weight loss is defined as 1–2 pounds per week. Losing weight at a faster pace could be a sign you're not eating enough nutrients. These restrictive eating habits often lead to a distorted relationship with food and other symptoms. Headaches, moodiness, constipation, and menstrual irregularities are just a few of the many red flags associated with rapid weight changes. Studies also link fast weight loss to long-term complications including gallstones, hair loss, diminished skin elasticity, and deteriorated lean muscle mass. A review published in the *British Journal of Nutrition* in June 2020 resolved the debate between fast and slow weight loss, noting the "beneficial effects of gradual weight loss, as compared with rapid weight loss, on body fat and resting metabolism." Healthy, slow weight loss prevails when it comes to long-term success and sustainability.

## Learn about Leptin

As mentioned in Chapter 6, leptin is a hormone in your body responsible for feelings of fullness. Leptin is secreted in response to eating food and sends a message to your brain that you had enough to eat and can move on to another activity. Yet, as you lose body fat, leptin levels can also decline. That is why you may notice increased hunger and appetite as you get closer to your target weight. Slow weight loss can minimize this effect and give your body time to adjust and adapt.

Aside from eating a strategic balance of high-fiber carbs, lean proteins, and anti-inflammatory fats that promotes satiety, eating at regular intervals, proper sleep, and moderate exercise will help. A sleep deficiency, in particular, can not only decrease circulating leptin, but also increase ghrelin, your appetite-stimulating hormone.

Ultimately, it is always important to respect and satisfy your hunger. Don't fight against it. Deprivation might accelerate weight loss, but it also backfires. Instead, take it slow and it will be a much more sustainable journey.

## Keeping a Food Journal

Keeping track of what you eat can be incredibly insightful and help you stay accountable. As part of the Core Three Plan, *I recommend you journal your food at least three days per week, or for at least the first three months of starting your journey.* Three days per week, including two weekdays and one weekend day, is enough to stay aware and assess eating habits throughout the entire week. It is also more manageable and realistic than tracking every single day. Food journaling is particularly beneficial if you feel like you're struggling. It can increase self-awareness and pinpoint problem areas, such as:

- **You have more cravings.** Food journals can help you determine if you're eating enough during the day or need to add in an additional serving of protein, fat, or non-starchy veggies that can help balance blood sugars, decreasing cravings.
- **Your progress is stalling.** Looking back at your food journals might reveal that you have been doing a lot more mindless snacking after dinner and on the weekends.
- **Your meal timing is off.** Food journals can show if you're eating dinner too late or eating more than you need in the evening.

Since writing down everything you eat can be time-consuming and is not the most natural way to navigate eating, 3 months at a time is often enough to benefit. However, it is always an accessible tool to use periodically as needed. Food journaling is not just limited to writing down what you've eaten. Including hunger levels and emotions can strengthen instinctive eating skills and help to distinguish between true hunger and emotional hunger. Here is a sample food record for guidance.

## Sample Food Journal

| FOOD + AMOUNT | TIME | SERVINGS (CARB, PROTEIN, FAT) | NON-STARCHY VEGGIES (3 MINIMUM) | FIBER (25G) | WATER (2–3 L OR 67–101 OZ.) | HUNGER 1–10 | EMOTION |
|---|---|---|---|---|---|---|---|
| 1 slice toast | 7:30 a.m. | 1 carb | | 3g | 20 oz. | 6 | Stressed |
| ⅓ avocado | | 1 fat | | 2g | | | |
| ½ cup tomato | | | x | 1g | | | |
| 5 oz. tuna | 1:30 p.m. | 1½ proteins | | 0g | 16 oz. | 6 | Distracted |
| 1 Tbsp. mayo | | 1 fat | | 0g | | | |
| 3 Wasa crackers | | 1 carb | | 6g | | | |
| 1 cup sliced pepper | | | x | 2g | | | |
| Apple | 4:00 p.m. | 1 carb | | 4g | | 4 | Tired |
| 1 Tbsp. almond butter | | 1 fat | | 2g | 12 oz. | | |
| 6 oz. chicken | 8:00 p.m. | 1½ proteins | | 0g | 16 oz. | 8 | Relaxed |
| 2 cups broccoli | | | xx | 10g | | | |
| 1 Tbsp. extra-virgin olive oil | | 1 fat | | 0g | | | |
| 2 Tbsp. grated cheese | | 0 | | 0g | | | |
| 2 cups green salad with vinegar dressing | | | xx | 2g | | | |
| 2% Greek yogurt | 9:30 p.m. | 1 protein | | 0g | 10 oz. | 5 | Tired |
| 1½ Tbsp. chocolate chips | | 1 flexible carb | | 0g | | | |
| Summary: | | 4 carbs 4 proteins 4 fats | 6 | 32g | 74 oz. | | Today I learned: I am grate-ful for: |

For extra support and accountability, you can send your journal to a friend or family member. You can also share it in the Core Three Facebook support group. Food journaling is a free and accessible tool—the ultimate behavior change instrument.

## What about Dining Out?

Dining out is not only allowed but necessary—it is a part of finding food freedom and living your life. Dining out provides the opportunity to socialize and connect by sharing a meal with others, which helps bring more satisfaction around eating. You can enjoy almost any cuisine when you focus on what a balanced plate looks like: ½ dish non-starchy veggies, ¼ dish protein, and ¼ dish starch. Fats are usually incorporated in sauces, marinades, dips, and dressings. This may not be an exact replica of your personalized servings, but it provides the necessary framework so that you can otherwise listen to your body. Use this dish method and the following additional guidelines for ordering in and dining out:

- **Don't arrive with an empty stomach.** On a scale of 1–10 (1 being full and 10 being ravenous) aim to be around a 6, not a 10. Ordering a balanced meal and eating mindfully is much harder on an empty stomach.
- **Start with a soup or salad.** Filling up on fiber-rich veggies before the main

course can help pace your eating, allowing you to recognize fullness and stop when you need to. If none of the soup and salad options look appetizing, lean protein–rich apps will also suffice.
- **Decide if you want a drink or dessert.** Compromising with yourself by choosing alcohol *or* dessert is the best approach to enjoying eating while still feeling good about your choices. Either can count as a flexible carb.
- **Drink up.** Have a glass of water when you sit down, and then keep rehydrating. We often confuse thirst and hunger, so staying hydrated can prevent overeating.

You always have the option to use your dining out as a weekly flexible meal. Remember, an occasional flexible meal is not a "cheat" meal—that term implies you're doing something *bad or wrong*. Instead, it's a chance to enjoy your favorite foods without overthinking it. Either way, dining out doesn't have to be a diet disaster. In fact, it is an important aspect that separates the Core Three Plan from other diets.

## Behavior Change Underlies Success

Creating long-lasting behavior change like implementing a healthy eating plan requires proper strategizing and a well-functioning design. The following strategies can help you maintain your success:

- **Be specific.** Eating more veggies, exercising more, and improving your relationship with food are all fantastic goals, but how are you going to get there? Measurable change requires a more detailed plan. Instead of "eat more veggies," try adding 1 cup of spinach to your smoothie in the morning, incorporating sliced tomato into your sandwich at lunch, or roasting broccoli to eat with your chicken and pasta at dinner. The more specific you are, the more successful you will be.

- **Keep it small.** Big dreams are great but can also be overwhelming. Instead of losing 20 pounds in 4 weeks, aspire to lose a healthy 1–2 pounds per week. The smaller you start, the more successful you will feel.

- **Find a replacement.** It is easier to substitute a behavior than to completely stop it. If you struggle with mindless munching after dinner, allow yourself a snack, but make it more nutritious. Creating healthier habits means forming new ones to replace the old ones.

- **Figure out the why.** Why do you want to improve your relationship with food and/or lose weight? Find a compelling reason so that it remains a priority.

- **Reward yourself.** We are programmed to want rewards for hard work. Plan non-food-related prizes— such as a night out with friends, a night in with a movie, or splurging on a new outfit—after you hit certain milestones. We push ourselves when we know there will be a positive outcome. Of course, the real reward is that you're taking care of yourself, but you should still celebrate all your successes, no matter how big or small.

- **Seek support.** When you're trying to lean out, you need people to lean on. While the most important praise comes from yourself, having others cheer you on and keep you honest can make a world of difference. Share your progress with others for positive feedback.

- **Join the Core Three Facebook group.** The Core Three Plan believes in the power of community. If you are someone who struggles to find support on your own, please join the Core Three Facebook group, a private, safe, and supportive place to share ideas, gain insight, and find inspiration. Access is free and unlimited.

Have the confidence that you can do whatever you need to do to get to where you want to be. Creating goals and achieving them is the best place to start. It will build your confidence and empower you to persevere. Understand that your goals might also transform over time, but your aspirations are what matters. In the remaining chapters, I will provide meal ideas and recipes to make this plan come to life!

**CHAPTER 12**

# Meal Plans

Meal planning is a self-care habit that makes healthy eating easier and more convenient. When you take the time to invest in yourself with meal planning and prepping, it continuously pays off. The best part is that by spending a little extra time up front, you save a lot of time (and money) later. Take all the hours you would normally use in a week on shopping, cooking, and cleaning, and condense them. *Designate just three days per week for planning, prepping, and cooking.* This routine will help bypass the urge to order in and will eliminate most healthy eating obstacles, creating a path of least resistance.

In this chapter, I will be sharing easy-to-follow meal-prepping guidelines to jump-start your journey. You will also find sample meal plans to exemplify what a 3- and a 4-carb day look like. For those who have various food preferences or follow specific dietary guidelines due to various health conditions, religions, or moral reasons, I am also including dairy-free, gluten-free, vegan, and kosher meal plans. You will also see the total protein, fat, veggie, and fiber servings for each day in the plans. These plans are here to guide you and offer suggestions on how to follow a personalized plan.

## Meal-Planning Guidelines

You can start with the meal plans in this chapter and then come up with your own using the Core Three formula. The meal plans do not need the same level of detail as the plans in this chapter. You will not need to cook a different recipe for each meal of the day. A few recipes per week can be doubled or tripled up so that you have enough meals for the entire week. There are also guidelines for dining out in Chapter 11 in case that better fits your lifestyle. Keep it simple and flexible. Most of the Core Three recipes can be tweaked, modified, and adjusted to fit your needs and preferences. Here are additional meal-prepping guidelines (not rules) to set you up for success:

- **Pin up your meal plan.** Whether it's the meal plans I provide or a plan you put together, writing it out and hanging it up on your fridge will help you stay focused. Always allow for flexibility and freedom of choice in case you're not in the mood for a particular meal that specific night. Like food journaling, writing out your meal plans can provide accountability.
- **Turn your fridge into a mini salad bar.** Eating a balanced and healthy diet is significantly easier when it's convenient. Nothing is more convenient then having all your carbs, proteins, fats, and non-starchy veggies prepared, chopped, cooked, and ready

for consumption. Just keep in mind that when vegetables are cut, they can spoil a bit sooner. Use that as incentive to eat them up right away or add them into a soup or smoothie.

- **Select protein that is already marinated or cooked.** If you really want to save time or you dislike cooking meat at home, you can buy your chicken, fish, tofu, and lean beef fully marinated or even cooked. Be realistic about what you're willing and unwilling to do. Although precooked proteins may contain unknown ingredients in the sauce, such as extra oil, sodium, and possibly sugar, it is better to eat it this way than not to eat enough protein.
- **Stock up on frozen and canned options.** Both frozen and canned foods will keep you well stocked when you don't have a chance to go to the store. The best canned foods include proteins like tuna, salmon, and sardines and veggies like asparagus, spinach, and beans.
- **Look into meal kits.** If you prefer even less work in advance, meal kits can be delivered to your home, providing recipe cards and all the ingredients you need to whip up a warm meal in minutes. Just make sure each meal has at least one serving of each macro—high-fiber carb, lean protein, and anti-inflammatory fat—unless you're saving the carb for a flexible carb later. You might not be doing it *all* yourself, but you should still be proud of your efforts.

## Nutritional Needs

Most of these plans are based on *3 carbs* per day—the core carb count—but there is also a *4-carbs*-per-day plan too. Some days illustrate a day that has carbs, protein, and fat equally balanced and portioned. Other days demonstrate what it will look like as you move to the next step involving meal plan liberation with portioned carbs and varying amounts of proteins and fats. You can take this next step whenever you feel ready. I suggest initiating this process around the 3-month mark—when most people have noticed significant results, and discovering food freedom becomes increasingly important. Eventually, and depending on how you feel, you may choose not to portion out at all, and simply eat according to your body's signals. Regardless, you always have the Core Three plan to fall back on when you feel like you need more structure again.

When using these plans, adjust up or down as needed to align with your daily goals. These samples are meant to guide you as you work on your relationship with food and body image, as well as permanent behavioral changes. If you choose to follow these plans exactly, understand that you must still make room for variables. Some days you'll find yourself hungrier than others. In that case, you might need to eat more! If you eat outside the plan, you're not cheating, and you certainly have not failed. It is simply your body's way of telling you that perhaps you need a little more fuel,

require some extra nutrients, or are just craving more variety. All these meals, except for snacks and flexible carbs, have a recipe, which you can access in Chapters 13–15.

The snacks in these plans are placed in between lunch and dinner, but you are free to consume them when it feels right. It's best to eat a snack when you know there will be more than 4–5 hours before your next meal. Because of that, snacks may be appropriate between breakfast and lunch, between lunch and dinner, or even after dinner. Let your hunger guide you, and adjust as needed. If you find yourself snacking more than necessary, ask yourself questions to determine if your hunger is truly physiological or just emotional and stress-related. There are some days where there is no snack listed. This would be more appropriate on days when your meals are spaced out by an average of only 4 hours or if you are simply not someone who snacks. Snacks are not mandatory, but they can help prevent overeating and keep blood sugar and insulin levels stable. They also offer an additional opportunity to hit all your carb, protein, fat, and veggie goals.

You will also notice flexible carb suggestions on certain days. These are also optional. You can enjoy them between meals, with a meal, or after dinner. No matter what, save flexible carbs for a time of day when you will enjoy and appreciate them most. As with the rest of the meal plans and snacks listed here, make them a mindful eating experience.

## Meal Plan 3 Carbs

| DAY | BREAKFAST | LUNCH | SNACK | DINNER | MACROS | FIBER |
|---|---|---|---|---|---|---|
| 1 | ½ cup unsweetened almond milk, Homemade Cinnamon Nut Granola, 1¼ cups fresh blueberries | Tuna wrap: Classic Tuna Salad (½ serving), La Tortilla Factory wrap | 1-oz. reduced-fat cheese stick Flexible carb: 1 oz. pretzels | Shrimp & Zoodle Pesto, ½ cup cooked whole-wheat spaghetti | Carbs: 3 Proteins: 3 Fats: 4 Veggies: 3 | 28g |
| 2 | Three-Ingredient Pancakes, 1 scrambled egg | Vegetarian Cobb Salad (½ serving) | 1 oz. reduced-fat cheese + ⅔ cup shelled edamame | Italian-Style Turkey Meatballs (½ serving), ½ cup cooked whole-wheat pasta, 1 cup cooked zucchini | Carbs: 3 Proteins: 3 Fats: 4½ Veggies: 4 | 25g |
| 3 | Banana Nut Oat Smoothie Bowl, 1 Tbsp. chia seeds | Breakfast-for-Lunch Bento Box | 2 oz. reduced-fat cheese | Very Veggie Lasagna, (½ serving) 2 oz. grilled chicken | Carbs: 3 Proteins: 3 Fats: 4 Veggies: 3 | 30g |
| 4 | The Green Machine Smoothie | Mediterranean Pasta Salad, 3 oz. grilled chicken | 3 Wasa crackers, 2 Tbsp. hummus | Chicken Spinach Artichoke Spaghetti Squash | Carbs: 3 Proteins: 3 Fats: 3 Veggies: 5 | 38g |
| 5 | Spinach & Cheese Egg Muffins, 2 cups fresh strawberries | Simple Salmon Croquettes, 2 cups mixed greens | 1 cup celery sticks, ½ Tbsp. peanut butter | Vegan Burrito Bowl | Carbs: 3 Proteins: 3 Fats: 3 Veggies: 5 | 48g |
| 6 | Matcha Protein Balls (2 servings) | Apple Goat Cheese Arugula Salad | 1 sliced pear, ½ cup part-skim ricotta cheese | Mexican Shrimp Chopped Salad | Carbs: 3 Proteins: 3½ Fats: 6 Veggies: 5 | 34g |
| 7 | Blueberry Waffles | DIY Spicy Poke Bowl | ½ cup sliced mango + 1 Tbsp. almond slivers | Herb-Seasoned Hearty Turkey Chili (½ serving), ½ cup roasted cauliflower | Carbs: 3 Proteins: 4 Fats: 3½ Veggies: 4 | 45g |

| DAY | BREAKFAST | LUNCH | SNACK | DINNER | MACROS | FIBER |
|---|---|---|---|---|---|---|
| 1 | Banana Nut Oat Smoothie Bowl | Balanced Bento Box | 1 cup sliced cucumbers, sea salt | Chicken Lettuce Wraps, ½ cup cooked brown rice | Carbs: 4 Proteins: 4 Fats: 4 Veggies: 5 | 34g |
| 2 | Gluten-Free Cinnamon Banana Pancakes | Kale & Quinoa Bowl | 2 oz. reduced-fat cheese, 2 Tbsp. almond slivers | Italian-Style Turkey Meatballs, 1 cup steamed spiralized zucchini Flexible carb: 5 oz. red wine | Carbs: 4 Proteins: 3½ Fats: 7½ Veggies: 4 | 25g |
| 3 | Vanilla Yogurt Mug Cake | Simple Tuna Salad, 1 whole-wheat pita | 1 cup sliced celery and carrots, 1 Tbsp. almond butter | Turkey Tomato-Stuffed Peppers | Carbs: 4 Proteins: 4 Fats: 4½ Veggies: 3 | 25g |
| 4 | Breakfast Brownie Bar, 1 apple | Arugula Salad Pizza | ¾ cup blackberries, 6 oz. 2% Greek yogurt | Mexican Casserole | Carbs: 4 Proteins: 4 Fats: 4 Veggies: 4 | 34g |
| 5 | Overnight Gut-Feeding Oats | Classic Chicken Salad, 2 Wasa crackers, 1 cup baby carrots | 1 apple | Zesty Grilled Fish Tacos, 2 cups mixed green salad | Carbs: 4 Proteins: 4½ Fats: 5 Veggies: 4 | 35g |
| 6 | Cinnamon French Toast (½ serving), 1¼ cups blueberries | Breakfast-for-Lunch Bento Box | 2 hard-boiled eggs, 1 oz. reduced-fat cheese, 2 Wasa light crackers | Hearty Chicken Minestrone Soup, 3 Tbsp. Parmesan cheese | Carbs: 4 Proteins: 4 Fats: 5 Veggies: 3 | 40g |
| 7 | DIY Gluten-Free Bagel, 2 oz. smoked salmon, 1 Tbsp. reduced-fat cream cheese | Chopped Chickpea Salad (½ serving) | 2 kiwis, 4 Brazil nuts | Shrimp "Fried Rice," ½ cup cooked brown rice Flexible carb: 1 oz. Lily's chocolate | Carbs: 4 Proteins: 4 Fats: 4 Veggies: 4 | 28g |

| DAY | BREAKFAST | LUNCH | SNACK | DINNER | MACROS | FIBER |
|---|---|---|---|---|---|---|
| 1 | Gluten-Free Banana Muffins, 2/3 cup fresh blueberries | Mediterranean Pasta Salad (½ serving), 4 oz. canned tuna, drained | Flexible carb: 1 ounce pretzels | Easy Chicken Veggie Soup, 2 Wasa crackers | Carbs: 3 Proteins: 3 Fats: 5 Veggies: 5 | 40g |
| 2 | Gluten-Free Cinnamon Banana Pancakes | Crispy Cheesy Cauliflower Pizza (½ serving), 1 cup roasted broccoli | 1 pear, 1 cup 2% Greek yogurt, cinnamon | Sesame Ginger Tofu & Veggies, ½ cup steamed brown rice | Carbs: 3 Proteins: 3½ Fats: 4½ Veggies: 3 | 25g |
| 3 | Cinnamon French Toast | Apple Goat Cheese Arugula Salad | 1 cup baby carrots | Air-Fried Fish & Chips | Carbs: 3 Proteins: 3 Fats: 5½ Veggies: 4 | 32g |
| 4 | Vanilla Yogurt Mug Cake | Plant-Based Burrito Bowl | 1 hard-boiled egg, 1 cup sliced cucumbers | Chicken Lettuce Wraps | Carbs: 3 Proteins: 3 Fats: 3 Veggies: 4½ | 25g |
| 5 | The Green Machine Smoothie (kosher protein powder) | DIY Spicy Poke Bowl | 1 oz. reduced-fat cheese | Black Bean Veggie Burger, 2 cups roasted broccoli, ½ sweet potato | Carbs: 3 Proteins: 4 Fats: 4 Veggies: 3 | 42g |
| 6 | Spinach & Cheese Egg Muffins, 2 slices sprouted grain bread | Cold Dill Salmon Salad, 1 cup sliced carrots and celery | 1 apple | Herb-Seasoned Hearty Turkey Chili | Carbs: 3 Protein: 4½ Fats: 3 Veggies: 4 | 37g |
| 7 | Blueberry Waffles | ½ serving Classic Tuna Salad, 1 cup sliced celery, ½ cup cherry tomatoes | 1 cup sliced red peppers Flexible carb: 2 Tbsp. chocolate chips | Zesty Grilled Fish Tacos | Carbs 3: Proteins: 3 Fats: 3½ Veggies: 4 | 38g |

| DAY | BREAKFAST | LUNCH | SNACK | DINNER | MACROS | FIBER |
|---|---|---|---|---|---|---|
| 1 | Vegan DIY Bagel, 1½ tsp. almond butter, 1 banana | Plant-Based Burrito Bowl | No Cow Bar | Sesame Ginger Tofu & Veggies | Carbs: 3 Proteins: 3 Fats: 4½ Veggies: 4 | 48.5g |
| 2 | Matcha Protein Balls (2 servings) | Kale & Quinoa Bowl | 3 clementines, 2½ Tbsp. pistachios | Tofu Lettuce Wraps (replace chicken with tofu) | Carbs: 3 Proteins: 3 Fats: 6½ Veggies: 5 | 27g |
| 3 | Blueberry Cinnamon Chia Pudding | Chopped Chickpea Salad | Smoothie: 1 cup unsweetened almond milk, 1 oz. vegan protein powder, 1 Tbsp. almond butter | Easy Veggie Soup (without chicken; 2 servings), ¼ cup nutritional yeast, 2 GG crackers | Carbs: 3 Proteins: 3 Fats: 4 Veggies: 5 | 58g |
| 4 | The Green Machine Smoothie (using 1½ oz. vegan protein) | Apple Goat Cheese Arugula Salad (without goat cheese) | 1 peach | Black Bean Veggie Burger, 2 cups mixed green salad | Carbs: 3 Proteins: 3 Fats: 3 Veggies: 5 | 35g |
| 5 | Overnight Gut-Feeding Oats | Simple Tofu Salad (replace tuna with tofu), 1 Tumaro's Carb Wise Protein Wrap | Smoothie: 1 cup fresh sliced strawberries, 1 oz. vegan protein powder, 8 oz. plant-based milk | Mexican Chopped Salad (remove shrimp and double up on black beans) | Carbs: 3 Proteins: 3 Fats: 5 Veggies: 4 | 40g |
| 6 | Vegan Kiwi Lime Parfait (with 2 Tbsp. vegan protein powder) | Balanced Bento Box (vegan version) | 2 cups cherry tomatoes | Hearty Minestrone Soup (without chicken) | Carbs: 3 Proteins: 3 Fats: 4 Veggies: 5 | 46g |
| 7 | Blueberry Cinnamon Chia Pudding | Mediterranean Pasta Salad (replace pasta with 1½ cups Palmini), ¼ cup nutritional yeast | None | Vegan Burrito Bowl | Carbs: 3 Proteins: 3 Fats: 4 Veggies: 6 | 58g |

| DAY | BREAKFAST | LUNCH | SNACK | DINNER | MACROS | FIBER |
|---|---|---|---|---|---|---|
| 1 | Vegan Kiwi Lime Parfait | Classic Chicken Salad, 1 cup sliced carrots and celery | 1 hard-boiled egg, 2 GG crackers | Vegan Burrito Bowl | Carbs: 3<br>Proteins: 3½<br>Fats: 4<br>Veggies: 3 | 50g |
| 2 | Vegan DIY Bagel, ⅔ cup mashed raspberries, 1 tsp. peanut butter | Simple Salmon Croquettes, 1 light English muffin | 2 dried dates | Hearty Chicken Minestrone Soup | Carbs: 3<br>Proteins: 3<br>Fats: 3<br>Veggies: 3 | 27g |
| 3 | Breakfast Brownie Bars (2 servings) | Cold Dill Salmon Salad, 3 Wasa crackers, 1 cup sliced red pepper | ⅔ cup grapes, 1 hard-boiled egg | Mexican Shrimp Chopped Salad | Carbs: 3<br>Proteins: 3½<br>Fats: 5<br>Veggies: 3½ | 30g |
| 4 | Blueberry Cinnamon Chia Pudding | Chopped Chickpea Salad | ONE PLANT Bar | Shrimp "Fried Rice" | Carbs: 3<br>Proteins: 3<br>Fats: 5<br>Veggies: 3½ | 47g |
| 5 | Homemade Cinnamon Nut Granola, 1 cup coconut milk yogurt, 1 tsp. honey | Balanced Bento Box | ¾ oz. HU chocolate | Zesty Grilled Fish Tacos, 2 cups mixed green salad | Carbs: 3<br>Proteins: 4<br>Fats: 5<br>Veggies: 3 | 37g |
| 6 | Three-Ingredient Pancakes, 1 hard-boiled egg | Cold Dill Salmon Salad, 3 Ryvita multigrain crackers, ½ cup baby carrots | Raw Rev Glo Bar | Easy Chicken Veggie Soup Flexible carb: 5 oz. red wine | Carbs: 3<br>Proteins: 3½<br>Fats: 5<br>Veggies: 3 | 34g |
| 7 | Cinnamon French Toast | DIY Spicy Poke Bowl | 1 apple, 2 Brazil nuts | Sesame Ginger Tofu & Veggies | Carbs: 3<br>Proteins: 3½<br>Fats: 5<br>Veggies: 4 | 33g |

## Meal Plan 3 Carbs—Gluten-Free

| DAY | BREAKFAST | LUNCH | SNACK | DINNER | MACROS | FIBER |
|-----|-----------|-------|-------|--------|--------|-------|
| 1 | DIY Gluten-Free Bagel, 2 oz. lox, ⅓ avocado | Kale & Quinoa Bowl | 1 pear, 1 oz. reduced-fat cheese | Very Veggie Lasagna | Carbs: 3 Proteins: 3 Fats: 6 Veggies: 4 | 31g |
| 2 | Blueberry Waffles | Vegetarian Cobb Salad | 1 cup fresh sliced strawberries, 1 cup 2% Greek yogurt | Mexican Casserole Flexible carb: 5 Hershey's Kisses | Carbs: 3 Proteins: 3½ Fats: 3½ Veggies: 4 | 40g |
| 3 | Gluten-Free Banana Muffins | Simple Tuna Salad, 1 cup sliced celery and carrots, 2 slices Udi's Gluten-Free Millet-Chia Bread | 1 sliced kiwi, 1 oz. reduced-fat cheese | Herb-Seasoned Hearty Turkey Chili | Carbs: 3 Proteins: 5 Fats: 6 Veggies: 3 | 26g |
| 4 | Spinach & Cheese Egg Muffins, 1¾ cups blackberries | Arugula Salad Pizza (replace wheat tortilla with gluten-free version) | 4 cups air-popped popcorn, 1½ tsp. extra-virgin olive oil, 2 oz. reduced-fat cheese | Shrimp & Zoodle Pesto | Carbs: 3 Proteins: 3 Fats: 4½ Veggies: 4 | 35g |
| 5 | Homemade Cinnamon Nut Granola, 1 cup 2% Greek yogurt, 1½ cups fresh raspberries | Zucchini Pizzas, ½ cup cooked whole wheat pasta | None | Turkey Tomato-Stuffed Peppers (½ serving) | Carbs: 3 Proteins: 3½ Fats: 4 Veggies: 4 | 37g |
| 6 | Vanilla Yogurt Mug Cake | Crispy Cheesy Cauliflower Pizza | 1 apple, 1 hard-boiled egg | Chicken Spinach Artichoke Spaghetti Squash | Carbs: 3 Proteins: 3 Fats: 5½ Veggies: 4 | 29g |
| 7 | Overnight Gut-Feeding Oats | Classic Chicken Salad, 3 cups mixed green salad | 2 clementines, 2 oz. reduced-fat cheese | Air-Fried Fish & Chips | Carbs: 3 Proteins: 3 Fats: 5 Veggies: 3 | 32g |

CHAPTER 13

# Breakfast Recipes

Within each recipe, you will see calculated Core Three servings and detailed nutrition facts including carbs, proteins, fats, fiber, sodium, and so on. It is important to note, the Core Three servings are based on the ingredients used and not the total nutrition facts. For example, if a recipe has 1 banana and 1 tablespoon of peanut butter the total servings would be 1 Core Three carb and 1 Core Three fat. If you only look at the total nutrition facts to calculate servings using the reference ranges provided in Chapter 3, you may not notice occasional discrepancies. For example, a recipe may have a total of 30 NET carbs yet is only counted as 1 Core Three carb. According to the reference range, 30 NET carbs would come out to 1½ Core Three carb servings. That is because the reference ranges are more useful when trying to calculate servings based on pre-packaged, prepared, or processed food products, not home-made recipes that have all the listed ingredients easily accessible.

That said, there is no perfect way to go about portioning out your meal plan. If you are using other recipes not included in this book you can use either method: calculating based on ingredients or calculating using reference ranges based on the total nutrition facts. There will only be a slight difference. What is the reason behind these discrepancies? Because you are consuming nominal amounts of carbs from protein- and fat-categorized foods, nominal amounts of proteins from carb- and fat-categorized foods, and nominal amounts of fat from carb- and protein-categorized foods. Non-starchy vegetables also add some extra grams of carbs to the totals as well. However, as long as you're paying attention to your body's signals and following your personalized daily servings of carbs, proteins, fats, and non-starchy veggies, the extras should not affect your health or weight management goals—especially since you're mostly eating nutrient-dense foods.

# DIY Gluten-Free Bagels

*If you enjoy having something doughy in the morning, this gluten-free, easy-to-make bagel is the perfect vehicle for your favorite nut butter or creamy spread. It takes minutes to make yet packs in plenty of fiber and essential nutrients like vitamin E, iron, omega-3s, and calcium. This recipe can introduce more variety into your morning breakfast rotation so you're never bored. You can substitute coconut milk yogurt for the Greek yogurt if you prefer. Enjoy with any spread or topping of your choice, like cream cheese, peanut butter, almond butter, eggs, avocado, lox, or hummus.*

1 large egg

½ cup 2% Greek yogurt

⅔ cup almond flour

¼ cup ground flax (flax meal)

1 teaspoon baking powder

⅛ teaspoon salt

¼ teaspoon "everything bagel" seasoning

1. Preheat oven to 375°F.
2. Crack egg into mixing bowl and combine with yogurt.
3. Add in flour, flax, baking powder, and salt. Mix well.
4. Spray doughnut pan with oil. Sprinkle in seasoning on bottom, and then add in dough. (If you don't have a doughnut pan, you can simply make four balls; roll out into thin, long rolls; and then shape into bagels. Spray tops with oil or brush with a raw egg, and then sprinkle on seasoning so it sticks.)
5. Bake for 12–15 minutes or until edges are lightly browned.

**CORE 3 SERVINGS**

0 carb
½ protein
1 fat

**YIELDS**
4 bagels

**NUTRITION FACTS
PER SERVING
(1 BAGEL)**

| | |
|---|---|
| Calories: | 195 |
| **Fiber:** | **4g** |
| Carbohydrates: | 7g |
| Sugar: | 2g |
| Protein: | 10g |
| Fat: | 14g |
| Sodium: | 241mg |

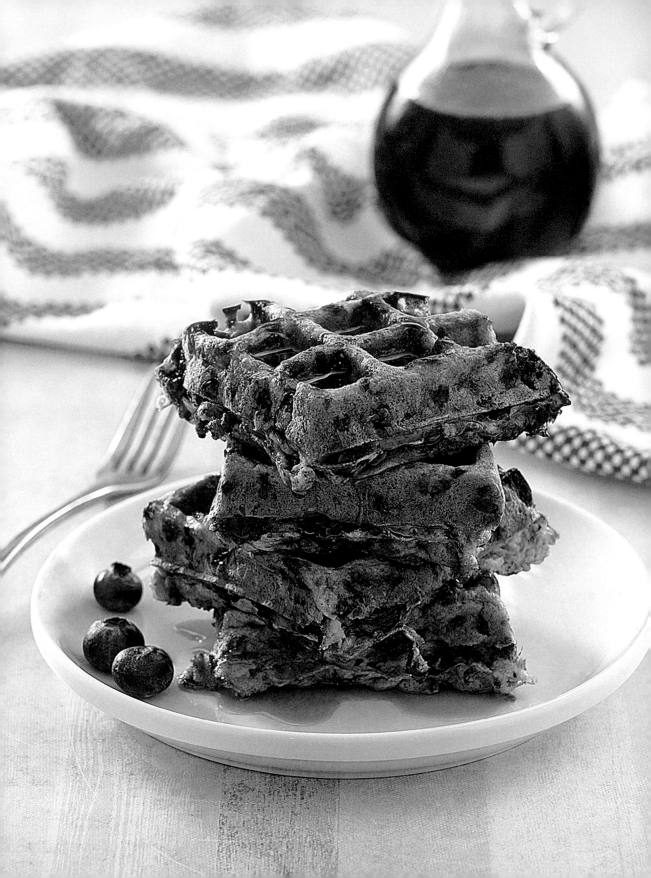

# Blueberry Waffles

*A hearty breakfast can go a long way when you have a demanding day. This recipe calls for high-fiber psyllium husk that is derived from the* Plantago ovata *plant's seeds and has prebiotic potential. This means psyllium can feed healthy gut bacteria, increasing probiotics and promoting a healthier digestive system to protect against gastrointestinal disorders. Psyllium can also increase the production of short-chain fatty acids, which studies show may increase your metabolism and fat-burning. Combining this gut-friendly ingredient with antioxidant-rich blueberries and protein-packed cottage cheese will keep you energized and satiated all morning long.*

1 cup frozen blueberries

1 tablespoon coconut oil

1 large egg

¼ cup cottage cheese

1 teaspoon vanilla extract

1 tablespoon psyllium husk powder

1 tablespoon vegan vanilla protein powder

½ teaspoon baking powder

1. Place berries in a microwave-safe dish and microwave for 1 minute.
2. Take out your waffle iron and coat the bottom and top with coconut oil so it's evenly distributed.
3. While the waffle iron is heating up, crack egg into a small mixing bowl.
4. Add in cottage cheese, vanilla extract, psyllium husk, protein powder, and baking powder. Mix well.
5. Pour batter over the waffle iron and lower the lid. Cook for 3–4 minutes, until slightly golden brown.
6. Let it cool for 1 minute, and then carefully remove from waffle iron. Once waffle is on the plate, finish with topping of your choice.

**CORE 3 SERVINGS**

1 carb
1 protein
½ fat

**SERVES**
1

**NUTRITION FACTS
PER SERVING**

| | |
|---|---|
| Calories: | 268 |
| **Fiber:** | **16g** |
| Carbohydrates: | 37g |
| Sugar: | 16g |
| Sugar Alcohol: | 1g |
| Protein: | 16g |
| Fat: | 7g |
| Sodium: | 524mg |

**OPTIONS**

You can swap the blueberries for strawberries and the cottage cheese for 2% Greek yogurt. If you don't have or don't use vegan protein powder, you can replace it with whey protein. The other option is to substitute the protein powder for 1 tablespoon of almond or wheat flour. For toppings you can choose a honey, peanut butter, or maple syrup drizzle.

**YIELDS**
4 bagels

**NUTRITION FACTS
PER SERVING
(1 BAGEL)**

| | |
|---|---|
| Calories: | 201 |
| **Fiber:** | **3g** |
| Carbohydrates: | 7g |
| Sugar: | 1g |
| Protein: | 6g |
| Fat: | 16g |
| Sodium: | 222mg |

## Vegan DIY Bagels

*If you're egg- and dairy-free or want to simplify the gluten-free bagel recipe even more, this one is for you. Combine a few household staples, bake, and then store in the fridge as an easy grab-and-go breakfast or afternoon snack. You can also make cinnamon-raisin bagels by adding in raisins, cinnamon, and vanilla extract for extra sweetness. Spread on your favorite nut butter or mashed avocado with a little sea salt or try tahini, peanut butter, almond butter, avocado, tuna salad, or hummus.*

1 cup almond flour

1 teaspoon baking powder

⅛ teaspoon salt

⅔ cup unsweetened coconut milk yogurt

¼ teaspoon "everything bagel" seasoning

1. Preheat oven to 350°F.
2. In a medium bowl, combine flour, baking powder, and salt. Mix well, and then fold in yogurt.
3. Spray doughnut pan with oil. Sprinkle in seasoning on bottom, and then add in dough. (If you don't have a doughnut pan, you can simply make four balls; roll out into thin, long rolls; and then shape into bagels. Spray tops with oil, and then sprinkle on seasoning so it sticks.)
4. Bake for 12–15 minutes or until edges are lightly browned.

## Matcha Protein Balls

*Matcha lattes are not the only way to acquire the benefits of anti-inflammatory, antioxidant-rich matcha green tea. These balls are quick, tasty, and full of nutritional value in every single bite. There's no cooking required—you just add a few simple ingredients to a bowl and roll it up into balls. Store them in the fridge and enjoy them as a snack or as a yogurt topping. Since matcha is a tea, it will have caffeine, so avoid consuming these too late in the day if you have a caffeine sensitivity. Omit the cinnamon if you like.*

2 tablespoons almond butter

1 teaspoon matcha green tea powder

1 tablespoon almond flour

1 tablespoon ground flax (flax meal)

1½ tablespoons vegan vanilla protein powder

⅛ teaspoon ground cinnamon

1. Add all ingredients to a bowl and mash together until well combined and smooth. Form into balls.
2. Refrigerate for 2–3 hours before eating so balls stay intact. Refrigerate leftovers for 1–2 weeks or freeze for a couple of months.

**CORE 3 SERVINGS**

0 carb
½ protein
1 fat

**YIELDS**
2 large balls or
4 small ones

**NUTRITION FACTS
PER SERVING
(1 LARGE BALL OR
2 SMALL)**

| | |
|---|---|
| Calories: | 139 |
| **Fiber:** | **3g** |
| Carbohydrates: | 6g |
| Sugar: | 1g |
| Protein: | 8g |
| Fat: | 12g |
| Sodium: | 27mg |

**SERVES**

1

**NUTRITION FACTS
PER SERVING**

| | |
|---|---|
| Calories: | 343 |
| **Fiber:** | **14g** |
| Carbohydrates: | 51g |
| Sugar: | 4g |
| Protein: | 13g |
| Fat: | 11g |
| Sodium: | 146mg |

## Overnight Gut-Feeding Oats

*Steel-cut oats are a little gritter than traditional rolled versions, but they are also slower-digesting—they don't raise your blood sugars as much as rolled oats. If you can handle the texture, they make for a valuable gluten-free grain that offers plenty of nutritional punch, such as soluble fiber, insoluble fiber, iron, and protein. You can enjoy this dish cold right out of the fridge or warmed up if you prefer. As mentioned in Chapter 4, when oats are eaten cold, or cooked and then cooled down, they contain more resistant starch that acts a prebiotic fiber, slowing down digestion and feeding probiotics in our intestines. That process promotes a healthy, strong, and resilient digestive tract. The special ingredient in this recipe is certainly sabja, or basil, seeds. They may be a new ingredient for you—mostly because they are often overlooked and not as well known as other seeds. Sabja seeds have more fiber than chia seeds but also provide iron, calcium, and antioxidants. They also absorb liquid a little faster. If you cannot find them online or in stores near you, you can replace them with chia or flax seeds. If you're not a fan of strawberries, frozen blueberries are an equally nutritious and delicious swap.*

¼ cup steel-cut oats

1 tablespoon sabja (basil) seeds

1 tablespoon chia seeds

½ cup frozen organic strawberries

¼ teaspoon vanilla extract

⅛ teaspoon ground cinnamon

⅔ cup unsweetened almond milk

1. Combine all ingredients in a glass bowl or jar.
2. Cover and store in the fridge for at least 4 hours or overnight. Seeds and oats will soak up milk and soften so mixture is ready to stir and eat in the morning.

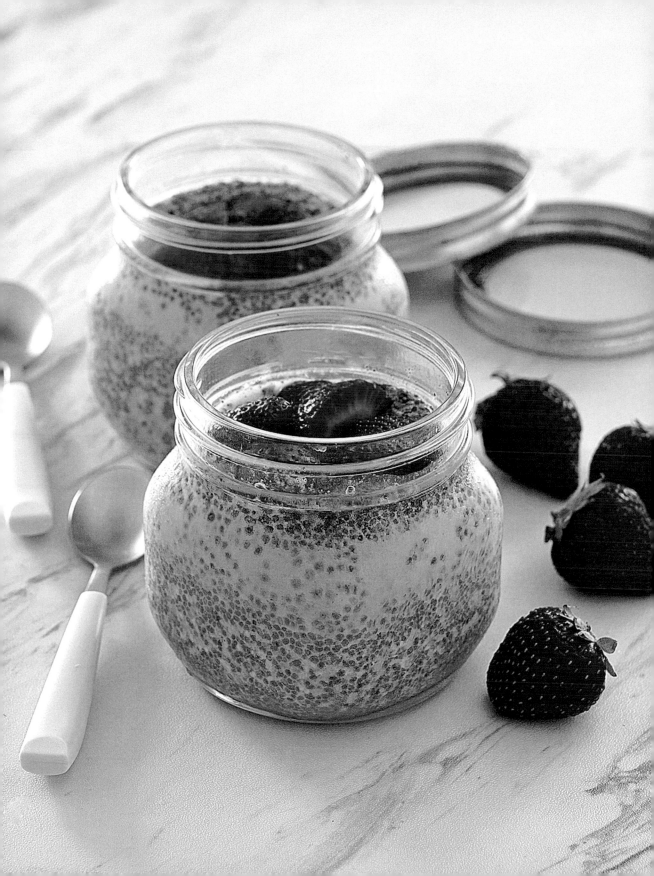

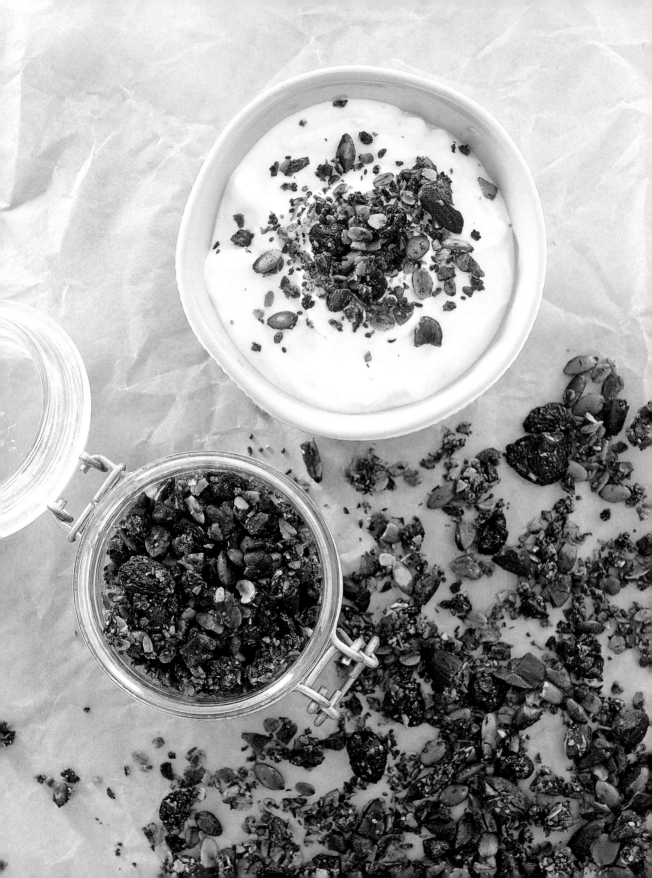

# Homemade Cinnamon Nut Granola

*This granola is a great crunchy topping for yogurt and is full of anti-inflammatory and high-fiber ingredients. Pumpkin seeds, in particular, are a frequently underrated nutritional powerhouse—a good source of heart-healthy potassium, mood-boosting magnesium, immune-supporting zinc, and blood-pumping iron. Studies also link pumpkin seed consumption with fighting inflammation and lowering blood sugars. You can enjoy this DIY granola dry or soaked in milk and experiment with different types of nuts, seeds, and dried fruit to suit your tastes.*

1/3 cup raw walnuts

1/2 cup unsalted pumpkin seeds (pepitas), shelled

1/2 cup raw almonds

2/3 cup dry rolled oats

1/4 cup Craisins

2 tablespoons ground flax (flax meal)

1 tablespoon chia seeds

1 large egg white

2 tablespoons coconut oil

1 teaspoon vanilla extract

1 teaspoon ground cinnamon

1 packet (2 teaspoons) stevia (optional)

1. Preheat oven to 400°F.
2. Place walnuts, pumpkin seeds, and almonds in a large zip-top bag and smash with any hard object to break apart. Do not overdo it, as you still want some chunks.
3. Transfer to a bowl and add in remaining ingredients. Mix well, and then spread over a parchment paper–lined baking sheet in an even layer to form a thin rectangle.
4. Cook for about 10 minutes or until edges are slightly browned. Let cool, and then break into pieces.

**CORE 3 SERVINGS**

0 carb
1/2 protein
1 1/2 fats

**YIELDS**
2 cups

**NUTRITION FACTS
PER SERVING
(1/4 CUP)**

| | |
|---|---|
| Calories: | 193 |
| **Fiber:** | **3g** |
| Carbohydrates: | 12g |
| Sugar: | 3g |
| Protein: | 6g |
| Fat: | 14g |
| Sodium: | 8mg |

**CORE 3 SERVINGS**

1 carb
1 protein
2 fats

**SERVES**
1

**NUTRITION FACTS
PER SERVING**

| | |
|---|---|
| Calories: | 357 |
| **Fiber:** | **8g** |
| Carbohydrates: | 35g |
| Sugar: | 16g |
| Protein: | 17g |
| Fat: | 17g |
| Sodium: | 247mg |

## Gluten-Free Cinnamon Banana Pancakes

*Pancakes are not just a treat for special occasions—this recipe can become one of your breakfast staples! The flax and almond flour replace traditional flour and are excellent sources of slow-digesting fiber and antioxidants. Per cup, almond flour has one-tenth as many net carbs as white flour, plus more iron, antioxidants, and anti-inflammatory fats. You can also replace the banana with 2–3 tablespoons of applesauce. Drizzle with a little maple syrup or, for extra protein, top with Greek yogurt and vanilla extract.*

1 banana

1 large egg + 1 egg white

2 tablespoons almond flour

2 tablespoons ground flax (flax meal)

¼ teaspoon baking powder

¼ teaspoon ground cinnamon

¼ teaspoon vanilla extract

1 teaspoon coconut oil

1. Mash banana in a medium bowl, and then add in egg. Mix well, and then add remaining ingredients except for oil. Stir until smooth.
2. Heat oil in a skillet over medium heat. Pour in batter to make about two 5-inch pancakes. Cook each side until sides start to bubble and begin to turn lightly brown, about 3 minutes per side.
3. Remove from pan, add topping of choice, and enjoy!

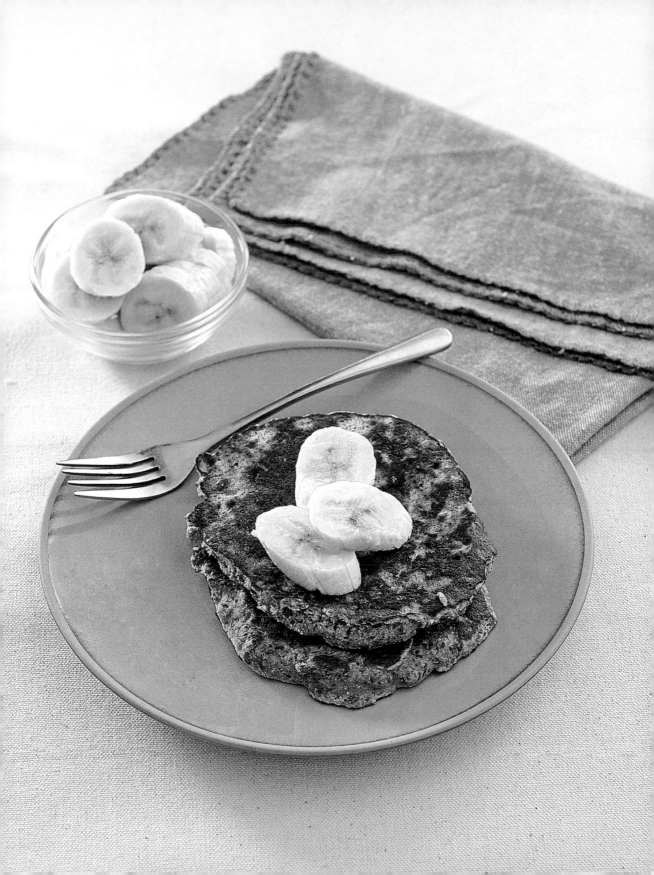

**SERVES**
1

**NUTRITION FACTS
PER SERVING**

| | |
|---|---|
| Calories: | 485 |
| **Fiber:** | **8g** |
| Carbohydrates: | 36g |
| Sugar: | 17g |
| Protein: | 17g |
| Fat: | 31g |
| Sodium: | 95mg |

# Three-Ingredient Pancakes

*You can never have enough three-ingredient recipes, especially in the morning when you need to get up and get out. This one includes a DIY sugar-free drizzle—that is also free of artificial chemicals—to replace traditional sugary syrups. If you want to make these into thinner pancakes or crepes, just add a bit of unsweetened almond milk to thin out the batter. For the vegan version of this recipe, simply swap the egg for a flax egg as explained in the directions, and for vegan or dairy-free, swap the butter for coconut oil. Top with fresh fruit like strawberries or raspberries.*

| *Pancakes* | *Pancake "Syrup"* |
|---|---|
| 1 banana | 1 tablespoon natural almond butter |
| 1 large egg | 2 tablespoons unsweetened almond milk |
| ¼ cup almond flour | ¼ teaspoon vanilla extract |
| 1 teaspoon butter | ⅛ teaspoon ground cinnamon |

1. For the Pancakes: In a small mixing bowl, mash banana, and then stir in egg and flour. Combine well.
2. Note: If replacing egg with a flax egg, mix 1 tablespoon ground flax with 3 tablespoons water. Let it sit in the fridge for at least 15 minutes so it thickens. (Pancake may not hold together as well as it does with egg, so you may need to add in an additional 2–3 tablespoons of almond flour as a result.)
3. Melt butter in a skillet over medium to high heat. Pour batter into skillet and cook for 3–4 minutes per side or until sides start to bubble or turn a little brown. Remove pancakes from pan and let cool.
4. For the Pancake "Syrup": In a small bowl, combine almond butter, almond milk, vanilla, and cinnamon. Mix well and pour over pancakes.

# The Green Machine Smoothie

*This is the one-stop shop of smoothies, incorporating all major food groups into a breakfast drink that will make you feel like a machine. Full of energizing nutrients and antioxidants, it should hold you over well until lunch. Blueberries are pure brain power, as they have been linked to enhancing mental acuity and delaying age-related cognitive decline—this is attributed to their relatively high antioxidant activity compared with other fruits. Normally, I recommend chewing your food instead of drinking it, since most people feel more satisfied after chewing, but when you blend specific foods together, it can be just as satisfying. If you're not into spinach, you can substitute kale, cauliflower, or carrots. You can also use flax or sabja (basil) seeds instead of chia seeds and choose any flavor protein powder you like.*

1 cup raw spinach

½ medium zucchini, sliced

¼ medium avocado

1¼ cups fresh or ⅔ cup frozen organic blueberries

1 tablespoon chia seeds

1 ounce vegan vanilla protein powder

¾ cup unsweetened almond milk

¾ cup water

Add veggies to a blender, followed by fruit and seeds, and then sprinkle protein powder on top, so when you blend, the powder doesn't get stuck to the glass. Fill with liquids and blend well!

**CORE 3 SERVINGS**

1 carb
1 protein
1 fat

**SERVES**
1

**NUTRITION FACTS
PER SERVING**

| | |
|---|---|
| Calories: | 254 |
| **Fiber:** | **13g** |
| Carbohydrates: | 49g |
| Sugar: | 21g |
| Sugar Alcohol: | 3g |
| Protein: | 19g |
| Fat: | 13g |
| Sodium: | 335mg |

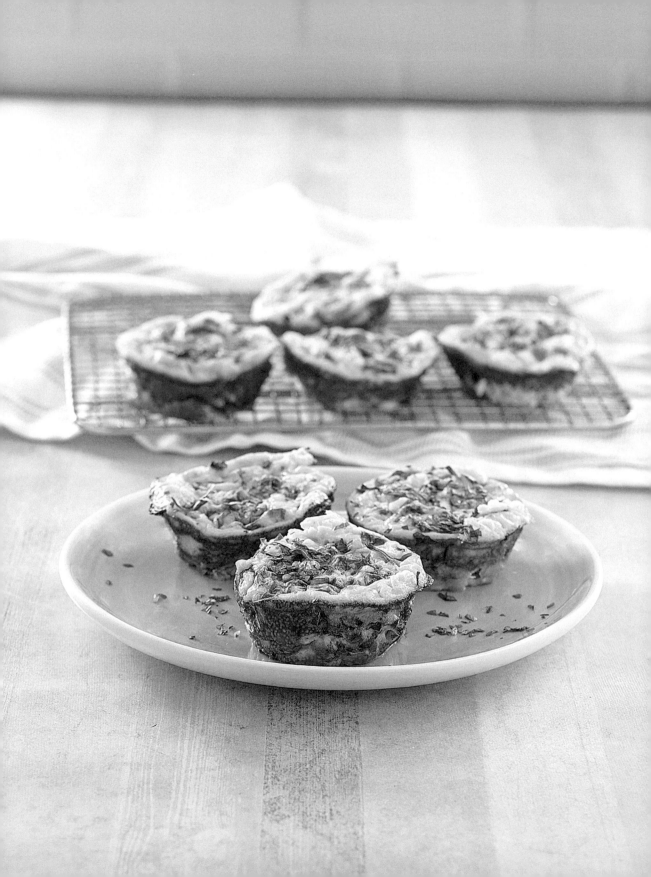

# Spinach & Cheese Egg Muffins

*Eggs are one of the easiest and most traditional breakfast protein sources. However, eating the same scrambled or hard-boiled eggs all the time can quickly get boring. Luckily, I have another option for you to start your day off happy and full. Adding in psyllium husk powder makes these savory muffins high in soluble fiber that can help regulate digestion and blood sugars. I also believe in eating the whole egg and not discarding the yellowy center. That is because yolks are nature's multivitamin—a great source of vitamins A, B, and D as well as iron, choline, and protein. You can store any leftovers in the fridge for 3–4 days and enjoy as a breakfast or afternoon snack. You can replace feta cheese with mozzarella, goat, or cheddar cheese. Top the muffins with chopped fresh parsley, if desired.*

**CORE 3 SERVINGS**

0 carb
1 protein
1 fat

**SERVES**
3

**NUTRITION FACTS PER SERVING (2 MUFFINS)**

| | |
|---|---|
| Calories: | 212 |
| **Fiber:** | **5g** |
| Carbohydrates: | 8g |
| Sugar: | 1g |
| Protein: | 17g |
| Fat: | 11g |
| Sodium: | 487mg |

6 large eggs

2 cups raw spinach, chopped

½ medium tomato, chopped

2 cloves garlic, minced

½ cup crumbled light feta cheese

2 tablespoons low-fat milk

1 tablespoon psyllium husk powder

⅛ teaspoon salt

⅛ teaspoon ground black pepper

1. Preheat oven to 375°F. Grease six muffin tin cups or line with paper liners.
2. Crack eggs into a large bowl and beat well. Add in remaining ingredients. Stir well, and then pour evenly into prepared muffin tin cups.
3. Bake for 15–18 minutes or until eggs are set or solid.
4. Serve immediately or refrigerate until ready to eat.

**SERVES**
1

**NUTRITION FACTS
PER SERVING**

| | |
|---|---|
| Calories: | 371 |
| **Fiber:** | **13g** |
| Carbohydrates: | 38g |
| Sugar: | 2g |
| Protein: | 14g |
| Fat: | 16g |
| Sodium: | 232mg |

# Cinnamon French Toast

*This recipe fits the bill for a comforting and balanced breakfast. French toast is traditionally high in refined carbs and sugars and low in fiber and nutrients. This version is the opposite of that: high in fiber and nutritious. The best part is that it takes only a few minutes to whip up and you can enjoy it on a regular basis. To make this recipe gluten-free, use a gluten-free whole-grain bread. Enjoy with the almond butter syrup in the Three-Ingredient Pancakes recipe earlier in this chapter or top with yogurt and fresh fruit. You can also enjoy a teaspoon or two of regular maple syrup or sugar-free syrup in moderation.*

1 large egg
½ teaspoon ground cinnamon
½ teaspoon vanilla extract
1½ teaspoons psyllium husk powder
1 tablespoon butter
2 slices sprouted grain bread

1. In a small mixing bowl, combine egg, cinnamon, vanilla, and psyllium husk. Beat well.
2. Melt butter in a skillet over medium heat.
3. While pan is heating up, carefully take each slice of bread and immerse each side in the egg mixture until saturated. Add to pan and let cook for a few minutes, until lightly browned (2–3 minutes per side).

## Gluten-Free Banana Muffins

*I love a tasty and easy muffin recipe. Full of flavor, fiber, and an array of nutrients, these muffins can be enjoyed by the whole family as a quick breakfast or satisfying snack. Ripened bananas offer plenty of natural sweetness on their own; there is no need to add additional sugar. If you like your muffins on the sweeter and softer side, you'll love how the vanilla yogurt enhances the taste and texture. This recipe includes chopped walnuts, but you can experiment by adding in fresh or dried fruit. You can also replace the 2 ripened bananas with ⅔ cup pumpkin purée and omit the vanilla yogurt if you like.*

2 ripe bananas

2 large eggs

⅓ cup low-fat vanilla yogurt

1 teaspoon vanilla extract

¼ cup chopped walnuts

2 tablespoons ground flax (flax meal)

2 cups almond flour

2 teaspoons baking powder

1. Preheat oven to 375°F. Grease eight mini-muffin tin cups or line with paper liners.
2. In a medium mixing bowl, mash bananas, and then add eggs. Mix well, and then add in yogurt, vanilla, and walnuts.
3. Combine flax, flour, and baking powder in a separate bowl, and then fold into wet ingredients until evenly combined.
4. Pour evenly into prepared mini-muffin tin cups. Bake for 25–30 minutes or until a toothpick inserted in the center is dry.

**CORE 3 SERVINGS**

½ carb

1 protein

4 fats

**SERVES**

4

**NUTRITION FACTS
PER SERVING
(2 MUFFINS)**

| | |
|---|---|
| Calories: | 528 |
| **Fiber:** | **9g** |
| Carbohydrates: | 28g |
| Sugar: | 10g |
| Protein: | 18g |
| Fat: | 38g |
| Sodium: | 45mg |

## Breakfast Brownie Bars

**YIELDS**

2 bars

**NUTRITION FACTS
PER SERVING
(1 BAR)**

| | |
|---|---|
| Calories: | 140 |
| **Fiber:** | **4g** |
| Carbohydrates: | 13g |
| Sugar: | 2g |
| Sugar Alcohol: | 1g |
| Protein: | 9g |
| Fat: | 9g |
| Sodium: | 71mg |

*There are plenty of delicious high-fiber protein bars available at stores. However, why buy them at the store when you can make them right at home with your own simple ingredients? Basic ingredients transform into a satisfying, rich, and balanced snack bar you can enjoy whenever the urge strikes. It can make for a grab-and-go breakfast, snack, or after-dinner treat. I used Orgain vegan chocolate protein powder in this recipe, but almost any protein powder will work here. You can also switch it up among almond, peanut, and cashew butter. If you want extra chocolate flavor, you can add in 1–2 tablespoons of chocolate chips and count it toward your flexible carbs for the day.*

2½ tablespoons protein powder

2 tablespoons peanut butter

1 egg white

2 tablespoons dry rolled oats

1½ teaspoons psyllium husk powder

½ teaspoon vanilla extract

⅛ teaspoon ground cinnamon

1. Preheat oven to 350°F.
2. In a small mixing bowl, combine protein powder and peanut butter. Blend well until smooth, and then add in egg white. Mix again until well combined, and then add in remaining ingredients. Give a final mix so all ingredients are evenly distributed.
3. Line a baking sheet with parchment paper and place mixture on top. Wet a fork or spoon and flatten out mixture evenly (wetting fork will prevent sticking). Shape into a thin rectangle. Bake for 10–12 minutes.
4. Remove from oven, let cool a few minutes, and then cut it in half along the length, about 2 inches by 5 inches (protein bar–shaped). Store in fridge and enjoy.

# Vanilla Yogurt Mug Cake

*While traditional cake is certainly not off-limits on Core Three, if you're trying to watch blood sugar or lose weight, this cake proves to be a worthy substitute. You can literally have your cake and eat it too—for breakfast, a snack, or an after-dinner-treat. The best part is it's easy to make and yields a single serving, so you can enjoy it to the last delicious bite. If you don't like bananas, you can substitute 2 tablespoons applesauce and half a chopped apple.*

1 large egg

1 egg white

2 tablespoons coconut flour

¼ teaspoon baking powder

2 tablespoons vanilla yogurt

1 banana

1. Add egg and egg white to a microwave-safe bowl or mug and whisk. Stir in flour, baking powder, and yogurt.
2. Slice banana and add half to the bowl with the other ingredients.
3. Microwave for 45 seconds. Stir, and then microwave for another 45 seconds.
4. Top with remaining banana and enjoy!

**CORE 3 SERVINGS**

1 carb
½ protein
½ fat

**SERVES**
1

**NUTRITION FACTS
PER SERVING**

| | |
|---|---|
| Calories: | 271 |
| **Fiber:** | **8g** |
| Carbohydrates: | 38g |
| Sugar: | 19g |
| Protein: | 15g |
| Fat: | 7g |
| Sodium: | 271mg |

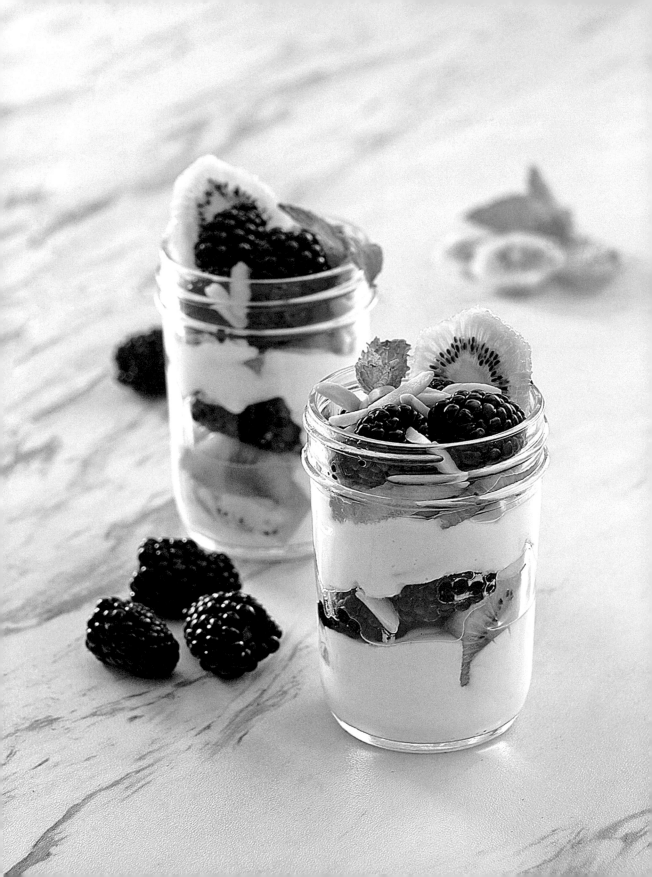

## Vegan Kiwi Lime Parfait

*Dairy-free eating doesn't have to feel restrictive, especially if you feel better limiting cow's milk. You can still enjoy all the pleasures that dairy eaters do. Take a classic yogurt parfait and jazz it up with vitamin C–rich kiwi, fiber-filled blackberries, and a crunchy almond topping. The mint and lime juice elevate this snack option to a whole new level, and fresh mint is a natural remedy for tummy troubles such as nausea and indigestion. You can also mix in 2 tablespoons of vegan protein powder for a protein boost. This will add 1 serving of vegan protein to the nutrition facts.*

1 (5-ounce) container coconut milk yogurt

1 teaspoon lime juice

1 kiwi, peeled and sliced

1 cup blackberries

2 tablespoons almond slivers

2 sprigs fresh mint

In a small bowl, combine yogurt and lime juice and mix well. Spoon half of yogurt into a medium Mason jar and spread evenly on bottom. Add in half of kiwi, half of blackberries, and half of almond slivers. Repeat layers once more and garnish with mint.

**CORE 3 SERVINGS**

1 carb

0 protein

1 fat

**SERVES**

1

**NUTRITION FACTS
PER SERVING**

| | |
|---|---|
| Calories: | 257 |
| **Fiber:** | **13g** |
| Carbohydrates: | 35g |
| Sugar: | 15g |
| Protein: | 6g |
| Fat: | 12g |
| Sodium: | 32mg |

SERVES
1

NUTRITION FACTS
PER SERVING

| | |
|---|---|
| Calories: | 409 |
| **Fiber:** | **8g** |
| Carbohydrates: | 48g |
| Sugar: | 24g |
| Protein: | 24g |
| Fat: | 17g |
| Sodium: | 252mg |

# Banana Nut Oat Smoothie Bowl

*Smoothies are not just for drinking. In fact, eating and chewing can be a lot more satisfying and signal your brain to register fullness. However, smoothies open up a world of opportunities to get in additional food groups and experiment with different flavors. As long as you maintain a balance of fiber, protein, and fat, you can enjoy any smoothie with a spoon and a bowl. Eating from a bowl also encourages a more mindful eating experience as it takes more time and requires more of your attention to consume. You can substitute steel-cut oats for the rolled oats; if doing so, blend the oats with the other ingredients instead of sprinkling them on at the end.*

1 banana
1 (6-ounce) container 2% Greek yogurt
1 cup unsweetened almond milk
⅛ teaspoon ground cinnamon
½ cup frozen cauliflower
2 tablespoons dry rolled oats
2 tablespoons chopped walnuts

Combine banana, yogurt, milk, cinnamon, and cauliflower in a blender. Blend well, and then pour into a bowl and sprinkle with oats and walnuts.

# Blueberry Cinnamon Chia Pudding

*Chia seeds are by far my favorite food recommendation. Considered a "superfood," chia offers a wide range of nutrients, including omega-3s, fiber, magnesium, calcium, iron, selenium, and B vitamins. In their natural state, these little black seeds have a tough exterior and are pretty flavorless, but when soaked in some liquids with other ingredients, they instantly become fun and delicious. Adding just 1–2 tablespoons of chia seeds per day can help fight constipation and inflammation. Berries are a leading source of antioxidants among the fruit family. Aiming for a few servings per week can help protect you from oxidative stress. For extra sweetness or flavor, you can add in a teaspoon of honey or maple syrup or a spoonful of almond or peanut butter.*

2 tablespoons chia seeds

1 cup frozen organic blueberries

½ cup unsweetened coconut milk yogurt

¼ teaspoon vanilla extract

¼ teaspoon ground cinnamon

Add all ingredients to a Mason jar or BPA-free storage container. Mix well and store in the fridge for at least 4 hours or overnight. The chia seeds will soak up the liquids and soften, turning into a pudding-like consistency.

**CORE 3 SERVINGS**

1 carb

0 protein

1 fat

**SERVES**
1

**NUTRITION FACTS
PER SERVING**

| | |
|---|---|
| Calories: | 247 |
| **Fiber:** | **13g** |
| Carbohydrates: | 35g |
| Sugar: | 14g |
| Protein: | 4g |
| Fat: | 11g |
| Sodium: | 27mg |

CHAPTER 14

# Lunch Recipes

Within each recipe, you will see calculated Core Three servings and detailed nutrition facts including carbs, proteins, fats, fiber, sodium, and so on. It is important to note, the Core Three servings are based on the ingredients used and not the total nutrition facts. For example, if a recipe has 1 banana and 1 tablespoon of peanut butter the total servings would be 1 Core Three carb and 1 Core Three fat. If you only look at the total nutrition facts to calculate servings using the reference ranges provided in Chapter 3, you may not notice occasional discrepancies. For example, a recipe may have a total of 30 NET carbs yet is only counted as 1 Core Three carb. According to the reference range, 30 NET carbs would come out to 1½ Core Three carb servings. That is because the reference ranges are more useful when trying to calculate servings based on pre-packaged, prepared, or processed food products, not homemade recipes that have all the listed ingredients easily accessible.

That said, there is no perfect way to go about portioning out your meal plan. If you are using other recipes not included in this book you can use either method: calculating based on ingredients or calculating using reference ranges based on the total nutrition facts. There will only be a slight difference. What is the reason behind these discrepancies? Because you are consuming nominal amounts of carbs from protein- and fat-categorized foods, nominal amounts of proteins from carb- and fat-categorized foods, and nominal amounts of fat from carb- and protein-categorized foods. Non-starchy vegetables also add some extra grams of carbs to the totals as well. However, as long as you're paying attention to your body's signals and following your personalized daily servings of carbs, proteins, fats, and non-starchy veggies, the extras should not affect your health or weight management goals—especially since you're mostly eating nutrient-dense foods.

# DIY Spicy Poke Bowl

*This delicious recipe is an easy way to re-create this fan favorite at home without having to handle raw fish, thanks to the omega-3-rich lox. This recipe also calls for edamame, otherwise known as soybeans. If you don't like lox, you can replace it with any type of protein such as chicken, hard-boiled eggs, tofu, or turkey slices. Add more or less of the sriracha, depending on how spicy you like the dish.*

### Bowl

1 tablespoon extra-virgin olive oil

2 cloves garlic, minced

2 cups riced cauliflower

2 cups spring lettuce mix

2 Persian cucumbers, diced

⅔ cup shelled frozen edamame, thawed

¼ medium avocado, diced

3 ounces wild lox (smoked salmon), rolled up and sliced down the width a couple times

### Dressing

½ tablespoon low-sodium soy sauce

1 teaspoon sriracha

1 teaspoon sesame seeds

1 teaspoon sesame oil

1. For the Bowl: Heat olive oil in a skillet over medium heat. Add garlic and stir for 1 minute. Toss in cauliflower and cook until softened, 5–10 minutes. Remove from heat and let cool.
2. Place lettuce in the bottom of a glass bowl, and then layer in cauliflower, cucumbers, edamame, and avocado. Top with lox.
3. For the Dressing: Mix together soy sauce, sriracha, sesame seeds, and sesame oil. Pour over top of bowl.

**CORE 3 SERVINGS**

1 carb
2 proteins
2 fats

**SERVES**
1

**NUTRITION FACTS
PER SERVING**

| | |
|---|---|
| Calories: | 579 |
| **Fiber:** | **17g** |
| Carbohydrates: | 40g |
| Sugar: | 13g |
| Protein: | 38g |
| Fat: | 32g |
| Sodium: | 2,155mg |

**NOTE**

This recipe is higher in sodium. If you have a history of high blood pressure, or need to watch sodium intake for other reasons, I recommend omitting the soy sauce or replacing it with coconut aminos: It is made from the sap of coconut trees and has a slightly sweeter and less salty flavor.

## Simple Salmon Croquettes

**SERVES
2**

**NUTRITION FACTS
PER SERVING
(2 PATTIES)**

| | |
|---|---|
| Calories: | 301 |
| **Fiber:** | **2g** |
| Carbohydrates: | 15g |
| Sugar: | 2g |
| Protein: | 35g |
| Fat: | 10g |
| Sodium: | 1,008mg |

**NOTE**

Keep in mind this recipe is higher in sodium. If you have a history of high blood pressure, or need to watch sodium intake for other reasons, I recommend cutting the salt out of the croquettes or the dipping sauce.

*Packed with omega-3s, wild sockeye salmon is one of the least contaminated (with PCBs) versions of salmon available. You can cook the croquettes in a pan with a tablespoon or two of olive oil or in your air fryer. Enjoy these croquettes with the optional dipping sauce, on top of a bed of greens, or with a carb of your choice like crackers, a whole-grain roll, or some fresh fruit. If you're gluten-free, replace the whole-wheat flour with the same amount of almond flour. If you prefer, you can swap in unsweetened almond milk yogurt instead of the full-fat Greek yogurt.*

*Salmon Croquettes*
1 (7.5-ounce) can wild sockeye salmon, drained
1 tablespoon lemon juice
1 tablespoon minced fresh parsley
2 tablespoons minced red bell pepper
1 large egg
¼ cup whole-wheat flour
⅛ teaspoon salt
¼ teaspoon garlic powder
1 tablespoon Dijon mustard
Olive oil spray

*Dipping Sauce*
¼ cup full-fat Greek yogurt
2 teaspoons lemon juice
1 teaspoon Dijon mustard
⅛ teaspoon salt
1 tablespoon chopped fresh parsley

1. For the Salmon Croquettes: Preheat oven to 400°F. Line a baking sheet with parchment paper.
2. Add all ingredients except oil spray to a food processor and pulse for 10–15 seconds. (If you don't have a food processor, you can add them to a mixing bowl and combine well.)
3. Remove mixture from processor bowl, form into four patties, and place on prepared baking sheet. Press down with fork or spoon. Spray with oil and bake for about 15 minutes.
4. For the Dipping Sauce: While croquettes are cooking, combine all sauce ingredients in a small bowl.
5. Once croquettes are done, serve with dipping sauce.

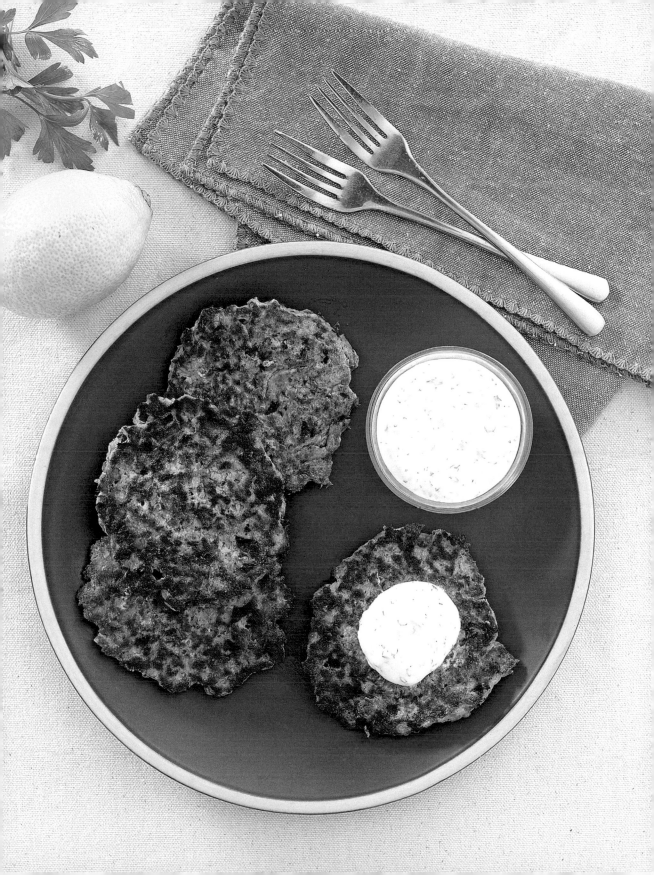

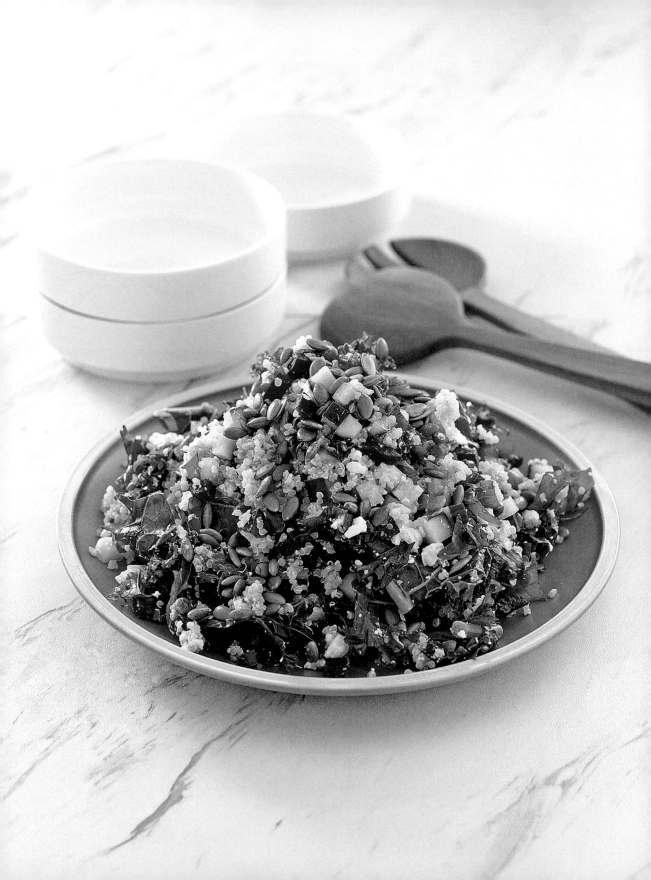

# Kale & Quinoa Bowl

*Everything tastes better in a bowl, and this combo is no exception. The key is to mix the kale with the quinoa right after it's cooked and still hot. It will wilt the kale, improving the kale's consistency and texture. While kale used to be reserved for garnishes, it has become one of the most widely recommended leafy green vegetables. Why? Kale is a nutrition superstar and a leading source of anti-inflammatory antioxidants; vitamins A, C, and K; fiber; and blood sugar–regulating manganese. Topping it off with toasted pumpkin seeds adds that satisfying crunch and so many additional nutrients to fight inflammation, nourishing your body.*

1 cup uncooked quinoa, rinsed and drained

2 cups water

3 cups raw chopped kale

1 tablespoon lemon juice

1 tablespoon extra-virgin olive oil

1 teaspoon Dijon mustard

½ medium cucumber, chopped

½ medium red bell pepper, chopped

1 ounce crumbled feta cheese

2 tablespoons toasted pumpkin seeds (pepitas)

1. Combine quinoa and water in a small saucepan and bring to a boil. Reduce heat to low, cover, and simmer until all liquid is absorbed and quinoa is softened, about 15 minutes.
2. Measure out 1 cup cooked quinoa and immediately add to a large glass dish or bowl along with kale. Store the rest in the fridge for later use.
3. Top with lemon juice, oil, and mustard. Stir well.
4. Once quinoa mixture has cooled down, add in cucumber, pepper, and cheese. Top with pumpkin seeds.

**CORE 3 SERVINGS**

2 carbs
1 protein
2½ fats

**SERVES**
1

**NUTRITION FACTS PER SERVING**

| | |
|---|---|
| Calories: | 575 |
| **Fiber:** | **10g** |
| Carbohydrates: | 57g |
| Sugar: | 9g |
| Protein: | 21g |
| Fat: | 30g |
| Sodium: | 421mg |

**TIP**

If you're not an animal-free eater, you can cook the quinoa in chicken broth for extra flavor.

# Simple Tuna (or Tofu) Salad

**SERVES**
1

**NUTRITION FACTS
PER SERVING**

| | |
|---|---|
| Calories: | 298 |
| **Fiber:** | **1g** |
| Carbohydrates: | 5g |
| Sugar: | 2g |
| Protein: | 28g |
| Fat: | 17g |
| Sodium: | 698mg |

*I love the versatility of canned tuna. It can be made so many ways and provides an exceptional source of omega-3s, as well as other essential nutrients. Enjoy it with crackers or bread or even stuffed into half an avocado. It is best to limit consumption of tuna to once per week due to its mercury content. However, if you choose canned light tuna instead of albacore tuna, it can be consumed up to three times per week, as it contains less mercury than albacore. You can replace the tuna with ⅔ cup firm tofu to make this recipe completely vegan.*

1 (5-ounce) can albacore tuna, drained

¼ cup shredded carrots

1 tablespoon extra-virgin olive oil

2 teaspoons lemon juice

2 teaspoons Dijon mustard

1½ teaspoons chopped fresh parsley

¼ teaspoon paprika

Add all ingredients to a small mixing bowl and mix well until evenly distributed.

## Classic Tuna Salad

*In my opinion, the best tuna salad is made with mayo. This was a constant in my house growing up, and it is also great for meal prepping so that you have a convenient ready-to-eat protein source in seconds. You can turn this into a tuna melt by spreading it on a slice of sprouted grain bread, topping it with a slice of cheese, and toasting in the oven at 400°F for 5 minutes.*

1 (5-ounce) can albacore tuna, drained

2 tablespoons mayo

1 hard-boiled egg

1 stalk celery, chopped

¼ cup chopped white onion

1 medium carrot, peeled and chopped

¼ teaspoon dried parsley

2 teaspoon lemon juice

¼ teaspoon ground black pepper

1 teaspoon ground flax (flax meal)

1. In a small mixing bowl, combine tuna and mayo. Mix well, and then add in egg and mash into the mixture.
2. Add all remaining ingredients and combine well.

**CORE 3 SERVINGS**

0 carb
2 proteins
2½ fats

**SERVES**
1

**NUTRITION FACTS PER SERVING**

| | |
|---|---|
| Calories: | 469 |
| **Fiber:** | **4g** |
| Carbohydrates: | 13g |
| Sugar: | 6g |
| Protein: | 35g |
| Fat: | 29g |
| Sodium: | 730mg |

# Chopped Chickpea Salad

**CORE 3 SERVINGS**

2 carbs
1 protein
2 fats

**SERVES**
1

**NUTRITION FACTS
PER SERVING**

| | |
|---|---|
| Calories: | 567 |
| **Fiber:** | **23g** |
| Carbohydrates: | 82g |
| Sugar: | 20g |
| Protein: | 23g |
| Fat: | 17g |
| Sodium: | 801mg |

*This leaf-free Mediterranean chopped salad is chock-full of fiber, plant protein, and antioxidants and is a wonderful meal-prep meal that you can keep in your fridge. Chickpeas are a nearly complete protein source, rich in all but one of the essential amino acids we need from our diet for growth, recovery, and repair. Chickpeas also provide a hearty dose of vital nutrients iron and magnesium. For that reason, and because it's easy to prepare, this is one of my go-to energizing lunches that I enjoy as often as possible. For additional protein, you can top it with shrimp, chicken, tofu, or hard-boiled eggs.*

### Salad
1½ cups canned chickpeas, drained and rinsed
1 cucumber, chopped
1 medium tomato, chopped
½ medium red onion, chopped
⅓ medium avocado, chopped

### Lemon Tahini Dressing
1 tablespoon tahini
1 tablespoon water
1 teaspoon lemon juice
⅛ teaspoon salt
⅛ teaspoon garlic powder
⅛ teaspoon dried parsley flakes

1. For the Salad: Mix all salad ingredients together in a serving bowl.
2. For the Lemon Tahini Dressing: Mix all dressing ingredients in a small glass bowl until well combined. Pour over salad and toss well so all vegetables are coated.

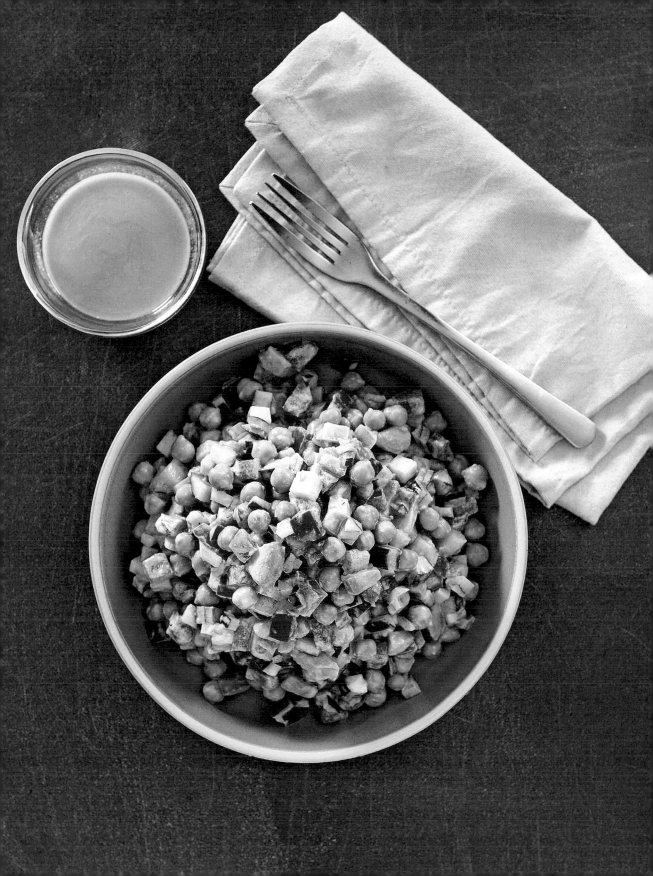

## Classic Chicken Salad

*If you're not a fan of tuna, chicken salad is a great alternative for a balanced, protein-packed lunch. This recipe combines a little sweet and a little salty, so you can have the best of both worlds. If you want to take the less traditional path, you can swap the mayo for full-fat or 4% Greek yogurt. This will add a bit more protein and gut-friendly probiotics. Otherwise, balance it out with a pita, crackers, and/or a crunchy salad.*

1½ teaspoons salt, divided
1 pound raw boneless, skinless chicken breast, cut into
    2½-inch cubes
½ cup halved grapes
2 tablespoons chopped walnuts
1 teaspoon ground black pepper
1 teaspoon garlic powder
6 tablespoons mayo
1 tablespoon chopped fresh parsley

1. Add 1 teaspoon salt to a pot of water and bring to a boil. Add chicken, reduce heat to low, and simmer for 2–3 minutes. Turn off heat, cover pot, and let chicken sit for 15–17 minutes while you prepare the rest.
2. In a large mixing bowl, combine grapes, walnuts, pepper, garlic powder, and remaining ½ teaspoon salt.
3. Once chicken is fully cooked, remove from pot and let cool. Add chicken and mayo to bowl with grape mixture and combine well. Garnish with parsley.

# Balanced Bento Box

*Lunchboxes are not just for kids. In fact, finger foods in a compartmentalized container can be incredibly convenient and healthy. Bento box lunches make it easy to keep your meals proportionate and balanced. You can purchase an adult-appropriate lunch box—or bento box—online and make bringing food to work a lot easier. Wash, cut, assemble, and you're ready to go. To make this recipe meat-free, swap the 4 ounces of turkey for 2 additional tablespoons of hummus.*

4 ounces turkey deli meat

2 tablespoons hummus

⅓ cup shredded carrots

⅓ medium avocado, sliced

1 cup cherry tomatoes, halved

1½ cups raspberries

Lay out turkey slices and top with sliced avocado. Roll up, and then assemble in bento-style lunch box along with remaining ingredients.

**SERVES**

1

**NUTRITION FACTS
PER SERVING**

| | |
|---|---|
| Calories: | 373 |
| **Fiber:** | **20g** |
| Carbohydrates: | 44g |
| Sugar: | 15g |
| Protein: | 27g |
| Fat: | 12g |
| Sodium: | 1,247mg |

**NOTE**

Keep in mind this recipe is higher in sodium. If you have a history of high blood pressure, or need to watch sodium intake for other reasons, I recommend limiting cured deli meats and using fresh sliced turkey or chicken breast instead.

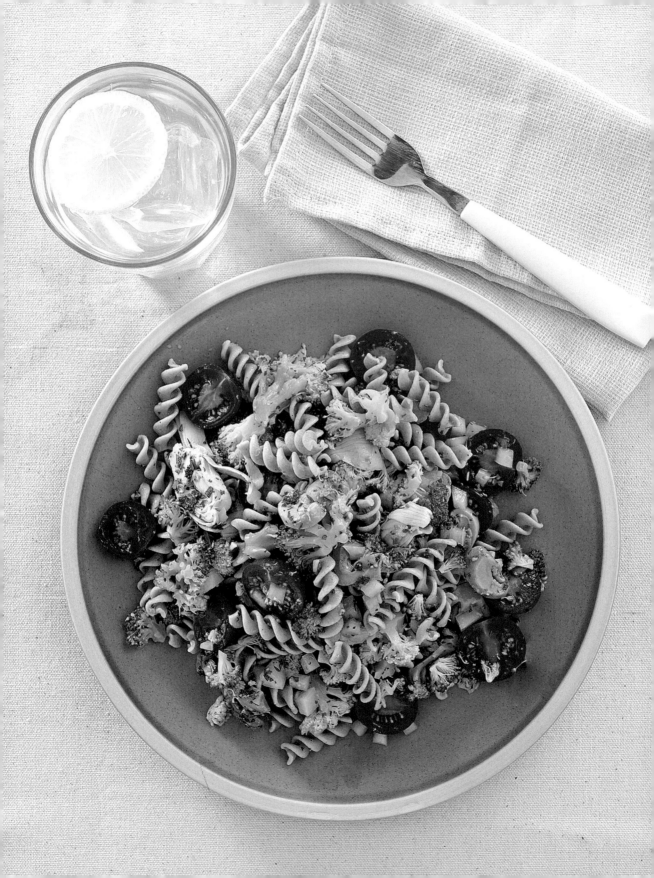

# Mediterranean Pasta Salad

*This is another easy meal-prep recipe that you can double or triple up so you have it ready-to-eat for the week. Top with whatever protein you prefer, like grilled chicken, canned tuna, baked tofu, turkey slices, or shrimp. If you're gluten-free, try brown rice, chickpea, or quinoa pasta instead of whole wheat. If you want to take out the carb serving completely, you can simply replace the pasta with 1½ cups of Palmini pasta, which is a non-starchy veggie made from hearts of palm. It comes in a can and must be drained and soaked in milk for 30–60 minutes before using.*

### Pasta Salad

½ cup cooked whole-wheat rotini pasta

1 cup cherry tomatoes, halved

1 cup chopped broccoli, steamed

½ medium yellow bell pepper, chopped

½ cup marinated mushrooms, sliced

3 artichoke hearts, canned in water, drained and sliced

2 tablespoons chopped fresh parsley

### Dressing

1 tablespoon extra-virgin olive oil

1 tablespoon water

1 clove garlic, minced

1 tablespoon red wine vinegar

1 teaspoon Italian seasoning

1. For the Pasta Salad: Combine all salad ingredients in a serving bowl.
2. For the Dressing: In a separate small bowl, combine all dressing ingredients. Pour dressing on top of salad.

**CORE 3 SERVINGS**

1 carb
0 protein
2 fats

**SERVES**
1

**NUTRITION FACTS PER SERVING**

| | |
|---|---|
| Calories: | 334 |
| **Fiber:** | **11g** |
| Carbohydrates: | 45g |
| Sugar: | 7g |
| Protein: | 10g |
| Fat: | 14g |
| Sodium: | 865mg |

## Breakfast-for-Lunch Bento Box

**CORE 3 SERVINGS**

1 carb
1 protein
2 fats

**SERVES**
1

**NUTRITION FACTS
PER SERVING**

| | |
|---|---|
| Calories: | 479 |
| **Fiber:** | **13g** |
| Carbohydrates: | 36g |
| Sugar: | 5g |
| Protein: | 27g |
| Fat: | 26g |
| Sodium: | 808mg |

*Mix up your lunch routine with breakfast-inspired staples like eggs and cheese. Experiment with different varieties of fresh fruit, crackers, and non-starchy veggies. Who needs Starbucks when you can have your own gourmet bento box from home? Okay, I went too far. We all need Starbucks.*

2 hard-boiled eggs, sliced
1 ounce reduced-fat cheddar cheese, cubed
4 light rye Wasa crackers
¼ cup guacamole
½ cup baby carrots
2 stalks celery, trimmed and sliced

Assemble all ingredients in bento-style lunch box.

# Apple Goat Cheese Arugula Salad

*Arugula is definitely an acquired taste worth acquiring. This nutritious leafy green veggie offers vitamins K, C, and A and potassium. When it's paired with creamy goat cheese and crunchy apples, the result is an ultimate taste trifecta. You can top the salad with grilled chicken breast, lean steak, or tofu for an additional protein boost.*

### Salad

1 teaspoon extra-virgin olive oil

½ medium red onion, chopped

½ cup cubed raw firm tofu

3 cups arugula

1 red or green apple, sliced

½ medium English cucumber, sliced into quarters

1 ounce goat cheese

### Dressing

1½ teaspoons lemon juice

1 teaspoon Dijon mustard

⅛ teaspoon salt

⅛ teaspoon ground black pepper

2 teaspoons avocado oil

1. For the Salad: Heat olive oil in a skillet over medium heat, and then add in onion. Cook until softened, about 15 minutes, and then add in tofu. Cook for another 5 minutes. Remove from heat and let cool.
2. In a serving bowl, combine onion and tofu with arugula, apple, cucumber, and cheese.
3. For the Dressing: In a separate small bowl, combine lemon juice, mustard, salt, pepper, and avocado oil. Pour dressing on top of salad and toss a few times to evenly distribute.

**CORE 3 SERVINGS**

1 carb
1 protein
2 fats

**SERVES**
1

**NUTRITION FACTS
PER SERVING**

| | |
|---|---|
| Calories: | 477 |
| **Fiber:** | **8g** |
| Carbohydrates: | 40g |
| Sugar: | 25g |
| Protein: | 20g |
| Fat: | 27g |
| Sodium: | 566mg |

**SERVES**
2

**NUTRITION FACTS
PER SERVING**

| | |
|---|---|
| Calories: | 313 |
| **Fiber:** | **6g** |
| Carbohydrates: | 15g |
| Sugar: | 7g |
| Protein: | 18g |
| Fat: | 20g |
| Sodium: | 459mg |

# Vegetarian Cobb Salad

*This hearty and delicious salad has all the best toppings, including avocado. Not everyone is avoca-devoted fan, but if you can keep an open mind, it is a wonderful source of anti-inflammatory fat, antioxidants, vitamin E, magnesium, potassium, and fiber. Traditional Cobb salads often include bacon, a high-pro-inflammatory, saturated fat–rich, processed meat. For that reason, it best enjoyed sporadically, and this Cobb salad concoction uses anti-inflammatory-packed homemade smoked almonds instead. If you truly cannot get over a meat-free Cobb salad, you can toss in smoked turkey, turkey bacon, or traditional bacon instead. Remember that processed meats such as saturated fat–rich pork bacon are best enjoyed as an indulgence one to two times per month. You can swap in goat cheese for the blue cheese and unsweetened almond milk yogurt for the Greek yogurt if you prefer.*

### Smoked Almonds

1 cup raw almonds

1½ teaspoons extra-virgin olive oil

¼ teaspoon paprika

¼ teaspoon chili powder

¼ teaspoon salt

### Creamy Herb Dressing

2 tablespoons lime juice

2 teaspoons avocado oil

⅓ cup 2% Greek yogurt

1 small clove garlic

1 tablespoon chopped fresh chives

⅛ teaspoon salt

⅛ teaspoon ground black pepper

½ teaspoon chopped fresh cilantro

*continued*

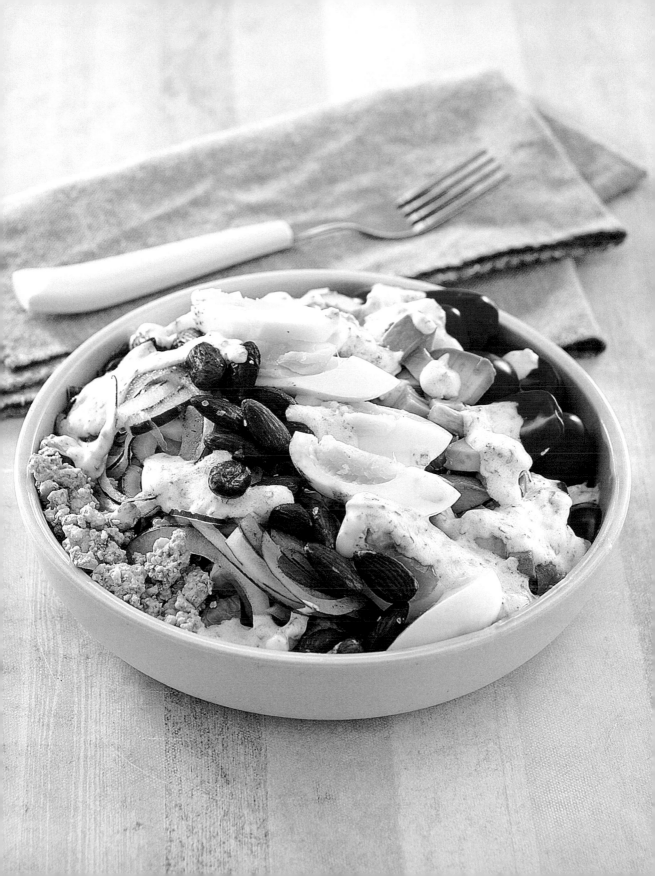

*Salad*

3 cups chopped romaine lettuce

2 hard-boiled eggs, quartered

1 ounce reduced-fat blue cheese, crumbled

¼ medium avocado, diced

1 cup cherry tomatoes, halved

¼ cup thinly sliced red onion

1. For the Smoked Almonds: Preheat oven to 375°F. Line a baking sheet with parchment paper. Combine almonds, oil, paprika, chili powder, and salt in a bowl. Mix well.
2. Lay almonds out on prepared baking sheet. Bake for 20 minutes. Remove from oven.
3. For the Creamy Herb Dressing: Combine all dressing ingredients in a food processor and blend until smooth. Cover and refrigerate for 30 minutes before serving. (Dressing can be stored in the fridge for up to 3 days.)
4. For the Salad: Place lettuce in the bottom of a serving bowl. Top with thin rows of egg, 2 tablespoons smoked almonds (reserve the rest for another use), cheese, avocado, tomatoes, and red onion. Drizzle dressing on top.

## Plant-Based Burrito Bowl

*This Mexican-inspired meal is entirely vegan with a healthy combination of fiber, plant protein, and fat. If you want to lower the carb total, replace the brown rice with riced cauliflower and the beans with tofu or grilled chicken. You can also use traditional shredded Mexican cheese instead of nutritional yeast, if you don't have nutritional yeast available or are not an animal-free eater.*

1 tablespoon extra-virgin olive oil, divided

⅓ cup diced white onion

2 cloves garlic, minced

½ cup steamed brown rice

⅔ cup canned pinto beans, drained and rinsed

1 tablespoon chopped fresh cilantro, plus 1½ teaspoons for garnish

2 tablespoons chopped scallions

1 medium tomato, diced

⅛ teaspoon salt

¼ cup nutritional yeast

1. Heat 1 teaspoon oil in a pan over medium heat, and then add in onion. Stir until translucent, and then add in garlic and sauté for 1 additional minute. Remove from heat and let cool.
2. Combine rice, garlic, onion, and beans in a serving bowl, and then add remaining 2 teaspoons oil. Add cilantro, scallions, tomato, and salt and mix well.
3. Top with nutritional yeast and garnish with additional cilantro.

**CORE 3 SERVINGS**

2 carbs
1 protein
1 fat

**SERVES**
1

**NUTRITION FACTS PER SERVING**

| | |
|---|---|
| Calories: | 462 |
| **Fiber:** | **13g** |
| Carbohydrates: | 63g |
| Sugar: | 6g |
| Protein: | 21g |
| Fat: | 15g |
| Sodium: | 627mg |

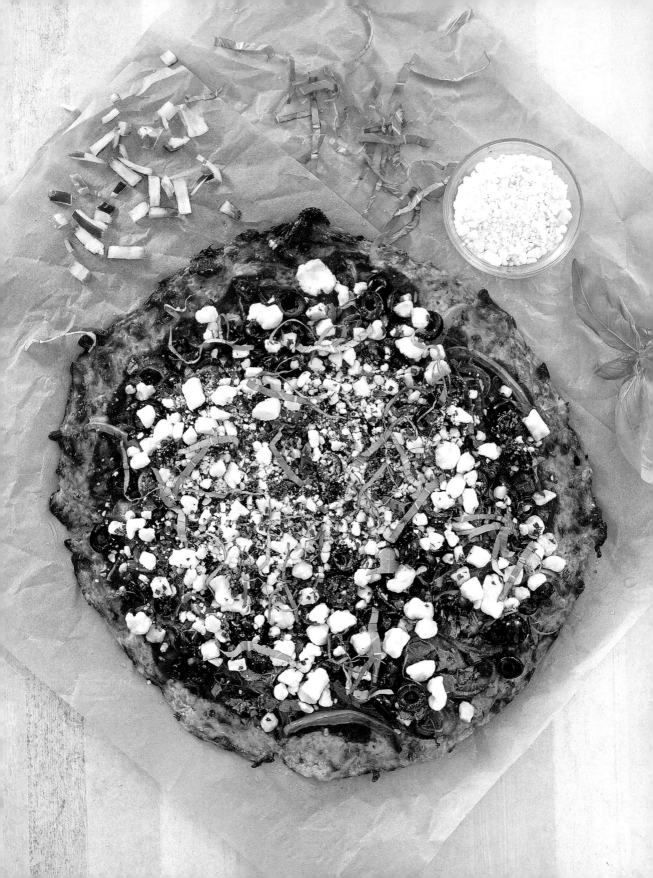

# Crispy Cheesy Cauliflower Pizza

*Nothing can quite replace traditional-style pizza, but if you want to maximize the nutritional value, why not make the crust with a high-fiber veggie? Cauliflower is incredibly versatile and can be used in a lot of recipes, thanks to its grain-like consistency and semi-neutral taste. The bonus is that cauliflower is a cruciferous veggie that also provides immune-balancing vitamin C, vitamin K for strong bones, energizing folate, and water retention–reducing potassium. You can play it safe with sauce and cheese or get more creative by piling on plenty of veggies and lean protein toppings.*

### Crust

4 cups riced cauliflower

2 large eggs

2 tablespoons grated Parmesan cheese

½ cup shredded mozzarella cheese

⅛ teaspoon salt

1½ teaspoons Italian seasoning

### Toppings

1 teaspoon extra-virgin olive oil

½ medium red onion, sliced

½ medium yellow bell pepper, sliced

½ cup tomato sauce

1 cup chopped raw spinach

¼ cup sliced black olives

½ cup crumbled goat cheese

1 tablespoon chopped fresh parsley

1 tablespoon chopped fresh basil

*continued*

**CORE 3 SERVINGS**

0 carb
1 protein
3 fats

**SERVES**
2

**NUTRITION FACTS PER SERVING (½ PIZZA)**

| | |
|---|---|
| Calories: | 417 |
| **Fiber:** | **6g** |
| Carbohydrates: | 20g |
| Sugar: | 8g |
| Protein: | 25g |
| Fat: | 25g |
| Sodium: | 815mg |

1. For the Crust: Preheat oven to 400°F. Line a baking sheet with parchment paper and line a medium bowl with a double or triple layer of cheesecloth.
2. Lay cauliflower on prepared baking sheet and bake for 15 minutes. Transfer cauliflower to prepared bowl. Let cool for 10–15 minutes, and then squeeze out excess liquid.
3. In a separate large bowl, combine cauliflower, eggs, Parmesan, mozzarella, salt, and Italian seasoning. Transfer to a baking sheet and spread into a thin layer. Bake for 20 minutes.
4. For the Toppings: While pizza crust is cooking, heat oil in a skillet over medium heat. Add onion and pepper and sauté until softened, about 10 minutes.
5. Remove crust from oven and top with tomato sauce, spreading sauce evenly in center of crust. Add onion, pepper, spinach, and olives, and then sprinkle on goat cheese. Return to oven and cook for another 10 minutes.
6. Remove from oven and let cool. Sprinkle with parsley and basil.

## Zucchini Pizzas

*Traditional pizza is certainly an option as a flexible meal, but you can still never have enough recipes that involve sauce and cheese. This easy-to-make zucchini-based dish also makes for a great adult- and kid-friendly snack or appetizer at social gatherings. It can also be replicated with other veggies like yellow squash, eggplant, and large portobello mushrooms.*

2 medium zucchini, sliced into ¼-inch-thick coins

1 tablespoon extra-virgin olive oil

⅛ teaspoon salt

½ cup marinara sauce

½ cup shredded mozzarella cheese

¼ teaspoon dried oregano

¼ teaspoon dried basil

¼ teaspoon garlic powder

1. Preheat oven to 400°F.
2. Place zucchini, oil, and salt in a large bowl. Mix well so that zucchini is evenly coated. (The other option is to spray both sides with olive oil and sprinkle with salt.) Lay zucchini on a greased or parchment paper–lined baking sheet. Bake for about 10 minutes, and then remove from oven.
3. Flip zucchini, and then spread on marinara sauce and sprinkle with cheese. Mix together oregano, basil, and garlic powder, and then sprinkle mixture evenly across zucchini.
4. Bake for another 5–8 minutes, until cheese is melted and slightly browned. Remove from oven, let cool for a couple minutes, and enjoy!

**CORE 3 SERVINGS**

0 carb
½ protein
1 fat

**SERVES**
2

**NUTRITION FACTS
PER SERVING
(½ PIZZA)**

| | |
|---|---|
| Calories: | 174 |
| **Fiber:** | **3g** |
| Carbohydrates: | 11g |
| Sugar: | 7g |
| Protein: | 8g |
| Fat: | 11g |
| Sodium: | 443mg |

# Arugula Salad Pizza

**CORE 3 SERVINGS**

1 carb
½ protein
1½ fats

**SERVES**
2

**NUTRITION FACTS
PER SERVING
(1 PIZZA/TORTILLA)**

| | |
|---|---|
| Calories: | 360 |
| **Fiber:** | **4g** |
| Carbohydrates: | 25g |
| Sugar: | 4g |
| Protein: | 16g |
| Fat: | 21g |
| Sodium: | 610mg |

**OPTIONS**

If you prefer your pizza with a kick, sprinkle on sriracha or hot sauce. You can also mix it up with different seasonings like cumin, garlic, black pepper, paprika, and parsley flakes. Or you can add in a tablespoon or two of red wine to enhance the flavor. After all, variety is the spice of life. Before serving, you can sprinkle each serving with ⅛ teaspoon red pepper flakes for an extra kick, if preferred.

*Arugula is an underrated leafy green that adds vitamins A, C, and K and calcium for stronger bones and a healthier immune system. Plus, this pizza is easy to make and versatile: You can replace the whole-wheat tortillas with gluten-free tortillas or swap the arugula with spinach or kale, if preferred. The egg is cooked just right when you follow the instructions exactly.*

1 tablespoon extra-virgin olive oil

½ medium red onion, sliced

¼ teaspoon salt, divided

2 cups arugula, coarsely chopped

2 large eggs

2 (6-inch) whole-wheat tortillas

2 ounces goat cheese

⅛ teaspoon red pepper flakes

1. Preheat oven to 375°F.
2. Heat oil in a skillet over low heat, and then add in onion. Sauté for 2–3 minutes, and then add in ⅛ teaspoon salt. Keep cooking until onion softens, about 5 minutes more.
3. Increase heat to medium and add in arugula. Cook for about 1 minute, and then add in remaining ⅛ teaspoon salt. Remove mixture from pan, and then crack both eggs into pan carefully so yolks do not break. Cook for 3–4 minutes, until bottoms are easy to scoop up with a spatula. Place eggs on a plate.
4. Arrange tortillas on a parchment paper–lined baking sheet and evenly distribute arugula and onion between tortillas. Sprinkle tops with goat cheese. Make a small nest in the middle of each tortilla and place 1 egg in each nest. Bake for 7–10 minutes, until eggs are cooked to desired doneness but tortillas are not burnt.

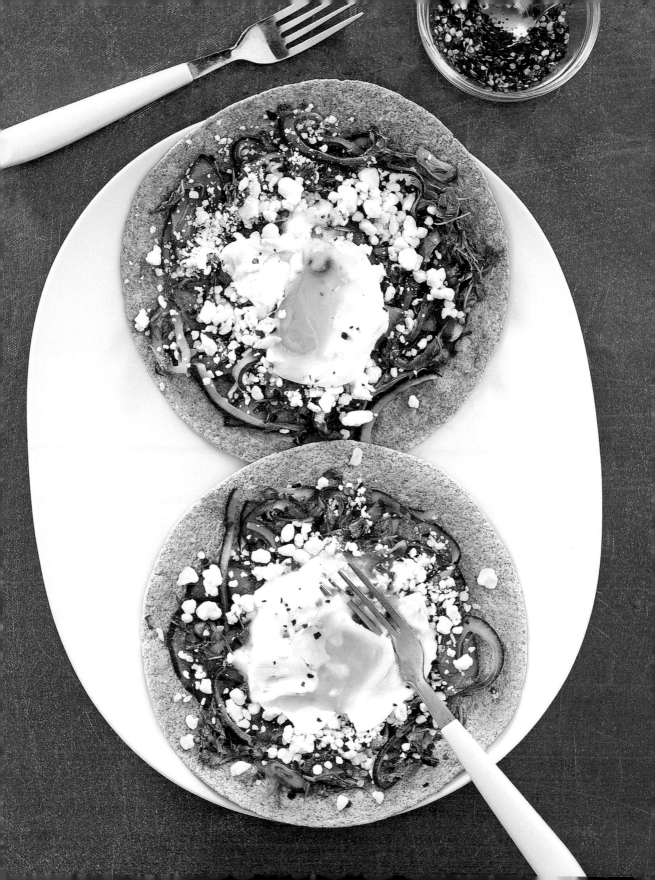

**SERVES**
2

**NUTRITION FACTS
PER SERVING**

| | |
|---|---|
| Calories: | 150 |
| **Fiber:** | **1g** |
| Carbohydrates: | 2g |
| Sugar: | 1g |
| Protein: | 22g |
| Fat: | 5g |
| Sodium: | 864mg |

# Cold Dill Salmon Salad

*Eating cold canned salmon is, without a doubt, the most convenient and affordable way to get in more anti-inflammatory omega-3 fatty acids. Since tuna is a higher-mercury fish, replacing it with canned salmon is a safer method to get in your three weekly servings of fatty, oily fish. This easy dish is delicious in a pita, with crackers, or over a fresh bed of leafy greens.*

6 ounces wild sockeye salmon

1 tablespoon Dijon mustard

1 tablespoon lime juice

¼ teaspoon salt

¼ teaspoon dried dill

2 stalks celery, leafy tips removed

1.  Drain salmon and move to a bowl. Add in mustard, lime juice, salt, and dill. Mix well.
2.  To serve, either chop celery and combine with other ingredients or spoon salmon salad into whole celery stalks and eat it that way.

# Dinner Recipes

Within each recipe, you will see calculated Core Three servings and detailed nutrition facts including carbs, proteins, fats, fiber, sodium, and so on. It is important to note, the Core Three servings are based on the ingredients used and not the total nutrition facts. For example, if a recipe has 1 banana and 1 tablespoon of peanut butter the total servings would be 1 Core Three carb and 1 Core Three fat. If you only look at the total nutrition facts to calculate servings using the reference ranges provided in Chapter 3, you may not notice occasional discrepancies. For example, a recipe may have a total of 30 NET carbs yet is only counted as 1 Core Three carb. According to the reference range, 30 NET carbs would come out to 1½ Core Three carb servings. That is because the reference ranges are more useful when trying to calculate servings based on pre-packaged, prepared, or processed food products, not home-made recipes that have all the listed ingredients easily accessible.

That said, there is no perfect way to go about portioning out your meal plan. If you are using other recipes not included in this book you can use either method: calculating based on ingredients or calculating using reference ranges based on the total nutrition facts. There will only be a slight difference. What is the reason behind these discrepancies? Because you are consuming nominal amounts of carbs from protein- and fat-categorized foods, nominal amounts of proteins from carb- and fat-categorized foods, and nominal amounts of fat from carb- and protein-categorized foods. Non-starchy vegetables also add some extra grams of carbs to the totals as well. However, as long as you're paying attention to your body's signals and following your personalized daily servings of carbs, proteins, fats, and non-starchy veggies, the extras should not affect your health or weight management goals—especially since you're mostly eating nutrient-dense foods.

# Mexican Shrimp Chopped Salad

*Spice up your salad routine with this fiery recipe. A balance of lean protein–rich shrimp, fiber-rich carbs, and anti-inflammatory fats rounds out your daily nutrients and your taste buds. If you don't eat shrimp, you can swap it for any type of fish, chicken, eggs, or tofu.*

### Salad

2 teaspoons extra-virgin olive oil

20 raw large shrimp, peeled and deveined

⅛ teaspoon salt

⅛ teaspoon ground black pepper

2 cups chopped romaine lettuce

½ cup canned black beans, drained and rinsed

⅓ cup frozen corn, defrosted

1 cup cherry tomatoes, quartered

¼ medium red onion, diced

¼ jalapeño, sliced

½ medium red bell pepper, chopped

### Dressing

2 tablespoons lime juice

1 tablespoon water

1 teaspoon avocado oil

1 tablespoon chopped fresh cilantro

1 clove garlic, minced

1. For the Salad: Heat oil in a skillet over medium heat. Season shrimp with salt and pepper, and then add to pan. Cook for 2–3 minutes per side, until fully cooked and pink on all sides. Remove from pan and let cool.
2. In a large bowl, combine remaining salad ingredients, and then top with shrimp.
3. For the Dressing: In a separate bowl or jar, combine all dressing ingredients, and then pour dressing on top of salad. Toss and enjoy!

**CORE 3 SERVINGS**

1 carb
1 protein
2 fats

**SERVES**
1

**NUTRITION FACTS PER SERVING**

| | |
|---|---|
| Calories: | 448 |
| **Fiber:** | **15g** |
| Carbohydrates: | 50g |
| Sugar: | 11g |
| Protein: | 32g |
| Fat: | 15g |
| Sodium: | 1,381mg |

**NOTE**

This recipe is higher in sodium. If you have a history of high blood pressure, or need to watch sodium intake for other reasons, I recommend cutting down the salt portion and switching to low-sodium canned beans.

**SERVES**
**4**

**NUTRITION FACTS**
**PER SERVING**

| | |
|---|---|
| Calories: | 570 |
| **Fiber:** | **8g** |
| Carbohydrates: | 44g |
| Sugar: | 12g |
| Protein: | 33g |
| Fat: | 27g |
| Sodium: | 775mg |

# Turkey Tomato-Stuffed Peppers

*This dish is fun to make and not very complicated. If you want to keep the carbs down, you can replace the brown rice with riced cauliflower. You can also swap the turkey for an equal amount of beef or chicken or 2 cups of black beans. This recipe is one the whole family will enjoy.*

4 large bell peppers, tops and cores removed

¼ cup extra-virgin olive oil

1 medium white onion, diced

4 cloves garlic, minced

1 pound 93 percent lean ground turkey

2 cups cooked brown rice

1 (14.5-ounce) can diced tomatoes

1 tablespoon tomato paste

1 teaspoon dried oregano

½ teaspoon salt

1 cup shredded light mozzarella cheese

1 tablespoon chopped fresh parsley

1 tablespoon chopped fresh basil

1. Preheat oven to 400°F.
2. Place peppers hollow side down in parchment paper–lined 13" × 9" baking dish and bake for about 10 minutes.
3. Heat oil in a large skillet over medium heat, and then add in onion. Sauté until soft, 5–10 minutes, and then add in garlic. Cook for 1 more minute, until garlic is fragrant, and then add in turkey. Cook until browned on all sides, breaking up turkey as you stir.
4. Add in rice, tomatoes, tomato paste, oregano, and salt. Reduce heat to low and simmer for 7–8 minutes. Remove from heat.
5. Once peppers are done cooking in the oven, stuff them with turkey mixture. Return peppers to the oven and bake for another 5–10 minutes, until peppers are tender.
6. Sprinkle cheese over top and return peppers to the oven for another 4–5 minutes, until cheese is melted. Garnish with parsley and basil.

# Italian-Style Turkey Meatballs

*We eat meatballs about once a week at my house. I blame it on my Italian husband, but really they're just an easy and reliable comfort food. If you've never tried making them with turkey, give it a whirl and you'll cut down on some additional saturated fat. However, if you prefer traditions, you can stick with beef and opt for grass-fed if possible. Enjoy these over a plate of whole-wheat, chickpea-flour, or brown-rice spaghetti.*

¼ cup grated Parmesan cheese

¼ cup bread crumbs

½ cup chopped red onion

4 cloves garlic, minced

¼ teaspoon salt

¼ teaspoon ground black pepper

¼ teaspoon dried oregano

1 pound 93 percent lean ground turkey

1 large egg

4 tablespoons extra-virgin olive oil, divided

1 (24-ounce) jar tomato sauce

¼ cup chopped fresh basil

1. In a large bowl, combine cheese, bread crumbs, onion, garlic, salt, pepper, and oregano. Mix well. Add turkey and egg and blend with your hands. Shape into 20 meatballs.
2. Heat 2 tablespoons oil in a large skillet. Add as many meatballs as will fit in one layer without crowding. Brown for 2–3 minutes, and then roll and brown for 2–3 minutes more. Transfer to a plate.
3. Add remaining 2 tablespoons oil to pan, along with remaining meatballs. Cook on all sides until lightly browned. (You can opt to bake meatballs at 400°F for 15 minutes instead of browning them in a pan.)
4. While meatballs are cooking, add sauce to a large pot and heat it up. Add browned meatballs to pot and stir gently so meatballs are fully covered. Cover pot and simmer for 15–20 minutes.
5. Transfer meatballs and sauce to a serving bowl and sprinkle with basil.

---

**CORE 3 SERVINGS**

0 carb
1 protein
2½ fats

**SERVES**
4

**NUTRITION FACTS PER SERVING (5 MEATBALLS)**

| | |
|---|---|
| Calories: | 473 |
| **Fiber:** | **2g** |
| Carbohydrates: | 17g |
| Sugar: | 7g |
| Protein: | 28g |
| Fat: | 31g |
| Sodium: | 966mg |

**OPTIONS**

If you want to shave off some carbs, you can instead pair the meatballs with sautéed spiralized zucchini, spaghetti squash, or shirataki (konjac) tofu noodles.

**NOTE**

Keep in mind this recipe is higher in sodium. If you have a history of high blood pressure, or need to watch sodium intake for other reasons, I recommend only enjoying on occasion.

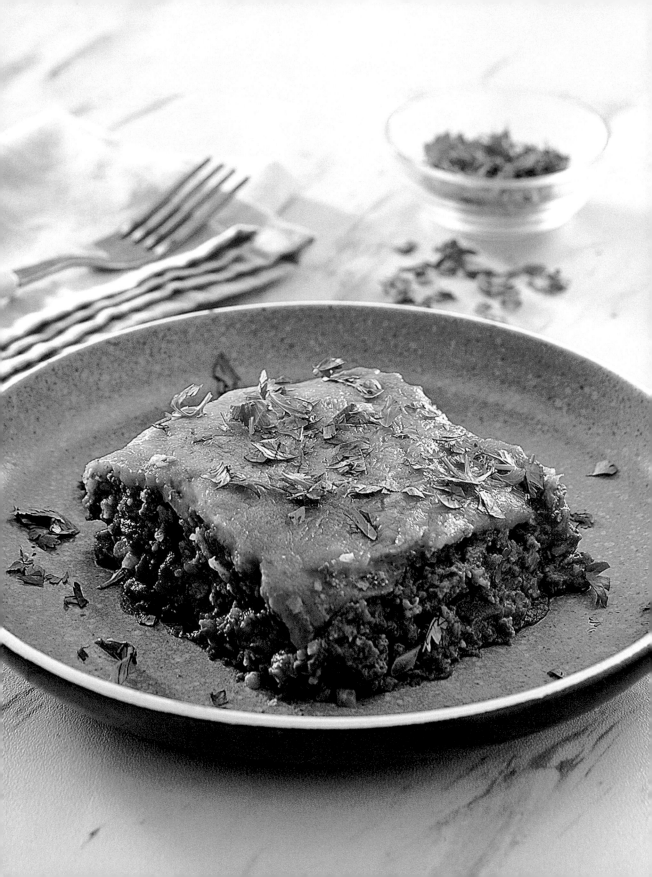

# Mexican Casserole

*This casserole is lower in carbs compared to traditional versions. However, if you want to go the more traditional route, you can replace the riced cauliflower with steamed brown rice and make it a heartier dish. Of course, the beans do introduce a small number of net carbs, as well as potassium, mood-regulating magnesium, blood-pumping iron, and plenty of gut-friendly soluble fiber that produces short-chain fatty acids, which directly stoke our metabolism. Grass-fed beef is not mandatory here, but remember that grass-fed contains more anti-inflammatory fats than conventionally raised cattle. Otherwise, it supplies a satisfying mix of lean protein, high-fiber veggies, and anti-inflammatory fats.*

**CORE 3 SERVINGS**

½ carb
½ protein
1 fat

**SERVES**
5

**NUTRITION FACTS PER SERVING**

| | |
|---|---|
| Calories: | 415 |
| **Fiber:** | **8g** |
| Carbohydrates: | 26g |
| Sugar: | 6g |
| Protein: | 31g |
| Fat: | 18g |
| Sodium: | 1,014mg |

**NOTE**

Keep in mind this recipe is higher in sodium. If you have a history of high blood pressure, or need to watch sodium intake for other reasons, I recommend only enjoying on occasion.

- 2 tablespoons extra-virgin olive oil
- 4 cups riced cauliflower
- ½ medium white onion, chopped
- 4 cloves garlic, minced
- 1 pound 95 percent lean ground beef
- 2 tablespoons taco seasoning
- 1 (16-ounce) can refried beans
- 1 cup chopped cherry tomatoes
- 1 (16-ounce) can diced tomatoes
- 1 cup reduced-fat shredded cheddar cheese
- 1 tablespoon chopped fresh cilantro

1. Preheat oven to 400°F.
2. Heat oil in a large skillet over medium heat. Pour in cauliflower and cook until tender, 5–8 minutes. Drain cauliflower and set aside.
3. Add onion to skillet, sauté until translucent, and then mix in garlic and beef. Cook until beef is browned, 7–10 minutes, and then sprinkle with taco seasoning.
4. Stir in beans, cherry tomatoes, and diced tomatoes and simmer for 15 minutes. Add cauliflower back to pan and cook for another 4–5 minutes.
5. Drain liquid from pan, transfer beef mixture to oven-safe casserole dish, and sprinkle cheese on top. Bake for 5–7 minutes or until cheese is melted. Garnish with cilantro.

# Black Bean Veggie Burgers

**CORE 3 SERVINGS**

½ carb
2 proteins
1 fat

**SERVES**
8

**NUTRITION FACTS
PER SERVING**

Calories:          210
**Fiber:             9g**
Carbohydrates:   22g
Sugar:              1g
Protein:           11g
Fat:                9g
Sodium:         446mg

*These DIY veggie burgers can be topped with salsa, hot sauce, or the Lemon Tahini Dressing from the Chopped Chickpea Salad (see recipe in Chapter 14). Serve with your favorite toppings like guacamole, tahini, organic ketchup, or cheese.*

2 (15.5-ounce) cans black beans, drained, rinsed, and patted dry

2 tablespoons extra-virgin olive oil

½ cup chopped red onion

½ cup chopped cremini mushrooms

2 cloves garlic, chopped

1 teaspoon chili powder

¼ cup ground flax (flax meal)

¼ cup almond flour

2 large eggs

⅓ cup grated Parmesan cheese

2 tablespoons chopped fresh parsley

2 tablespoons tomato paste

¼ teaspoon salt

⅛ teaspoon ground black pepper

1. Preheat oven to 325°F.
2. Spread beans evenly on a parchment paper–lined baking sheet and bake for 15 minutes, until slightly dried out.
3. While beans are baking, heat oil in a skillet over medium heat. Add in onion and cook until onion softens, about 5 minutes. Add in mushrooms and garlic and cook for 5–6 minutes. Gently blot some of the moisture out.
4. Place mushroom-onion mixture in a large bowl or in a food processor and add all remaining ingredients. Stir or pulse everything together, and then add the beans. Mash with a fork or pulse the mixture, leaving some larger chunks of beans.
5. Form into eight small patties and place on a parchment paper–lined baking sheet. Increase oven temperature to 375°F and bake for 10 minutes on each side, 20 minutes total. Refrigerate leftovers for up to 5 days or freeze.

# Shrimp & Zoodle Pesto

*A great pesto recipe can transform any dish from basic to gourmet. Pesto can be higher in fat, but it contains healthy fats that fight inflammation and help you keep you satiated. If you don't like spiralized zucchini, you can also spiralize yellow squash, use spaghetti squash, or incorporate whole-wheat spaghetti instead.*

**CORE 3 SERVINGS**

0 carb
1 protein
1½ fats

**SERVES**
4

**NUTRITION FACTS
PER SERVING**

| | |
|---|---|
| Calories: | 307 |
| **Fiber:** | **2g** |
| Carbohydrates: | 8g |
| Sugar: | 3g |
| Protein: | 20g |
| Fat: | 21g |
| Sodium: | 838mg |

**TIP**

To save time, purchase pre-spiralized zucchini if you don't want to spiralize it yourself.

### Pesto

¼ cup pine nuts

½ cup stemmed basil leaves

½ cup stemmed baby spinach

1 clove garlic

1 tablespoon lemon juice

¼ cup grated Parmesan cheese

2 tablespoons extra-virgin olive oil

### Shrimp and Zoodles

2 tablespoons extra-virgin olive oil, divided

1 pound raw shrimp, peeled and deveined

⅛ teaspoon salt

¼ teaspoon ground black pepper

1 tablespoon lemon juice

2 cloves garlic, chopped

4 cups raw spiralized zucchini

1. For the Pesto: Add pine nuts, basil, spinach, and garlic to a food processor and pulse until finely ground. Add lemon juice and cheese. With the machine running slowly, pour in oil and process until smooth. Set aside.

2. For the Shrimp and Zoodles: Heat 1 tablespoon oil in a large skillet over medium heat. Season shrimp with salt, pepper, and lemon juice, and then add to pan and cook for 2–3 minutes per side. Remove from pan.

3. Add remaining 1 tablespoon oil to pan and add in garlic. Cook for 1 minute, until fragrant, and then add in zucchini. Cook for 7–8 minutes or to your desired doneness. Transfer zucchini to a large bowl.

4. Top zucchini with shrimp and pesto. Mix well and enjoy.

## Chicken Lettuce Wraps

**CORE 3 SERVINGS**

0 carb
1 protein
1 fat

**SERVES**
4

**NUTRITION FACTS
PER SERVING**

| | |
|---|---|
| Calories: | 258 |
| **Fiber:** | **3g** |
| Carbohydrates: | 12g |
| Sugar: | 6g |
| Protein: | 26g |
| Fat: | 12g |
| Sodium: | 503mg |

**OPTIONS**

If you don't have fresh ginger, you can use ½ teaspoon of ground ginger instead and still retain most of the health benefits. To make this meal meat-free, simply swap out the chicken for 3 cups of firm tofu. You can also replace the Bibb lettuce with endive. Besides lettuce wraps, you can also enjoy the chicken/tofu and carrots over brown rice, riced cauliflower, or any veggie of choice.

*This recipe incorporates plenty of valuable ingredients into your diet that offer an abundance of antioxidants and anti-inflammatory properties. Studies show ginger can improve digestion issues, including nausea during pregnancy; reduce inflammation; protect against certain cancers; and reduce risk of diabetes and heart disease.*

**Pickled Carrots**

2 cups shredded carrots

1 tablespoon honey

⅓ cup unseasoned rice vinegar

**Wraps**

1 pound raw boneless, skinless chicken breast

1½ scallions, chopped

4 cloves garlic, minced

2 teaspoons minced fresh ginger

¼ cup low-sodium soy sauce

2 tablespoons coconut oil

1 head Bibb lettuce

1 teaspoon sriracha

**Sauce**

1 tablespoon sesame oil

2 tablespoons low-sodium soy sauce

½ scallion, chopped

1 clove garlic, minced

1½ teaspoons chopped fresh parsley

1 tablespoon sesame seeds

1. For the Pickled Carrots: In a medium bowl, combine carrots, honey, and vinegar. Let marinate in fridge while preparing the rest.
2. For the Wraps: Chop chicken into pieces and add to a large zip-top bag with scallions, garlic cloves, ginger, and soy sauce. Let marinate in fridge for 20–30 minutes.
3. Heat coconut oil in a skillet over medium heat. Add in chicken and cook for about 15 minutes, until all sides are browned and inside temperature reaches 165°F.
4. Remove from heat. Spoon chicken mixture into leaves of lettuce. Top with sriracha.
5. For the Sauce: Combine all sauce ingredients in a bowl and stir well.
6. Top wraps with pickled carrots and sauce.

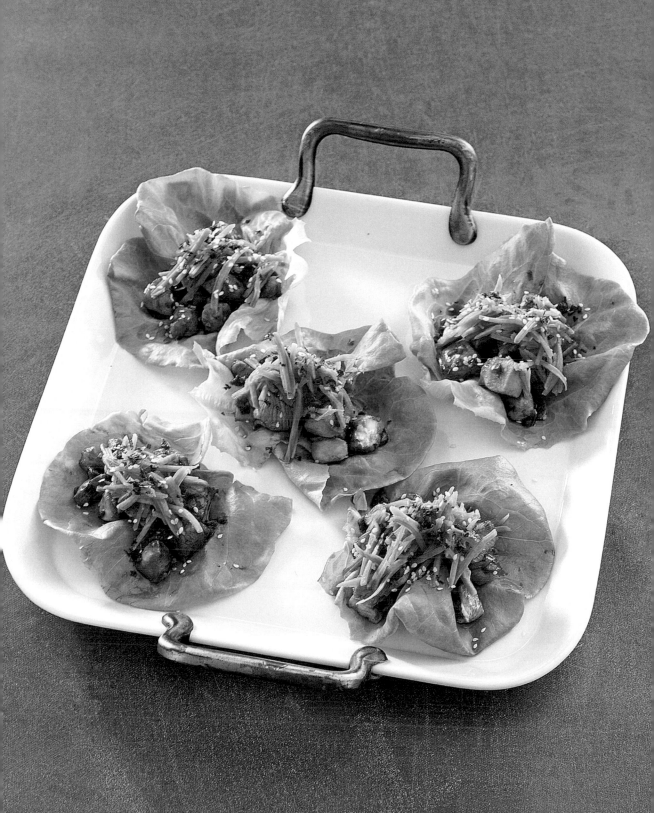

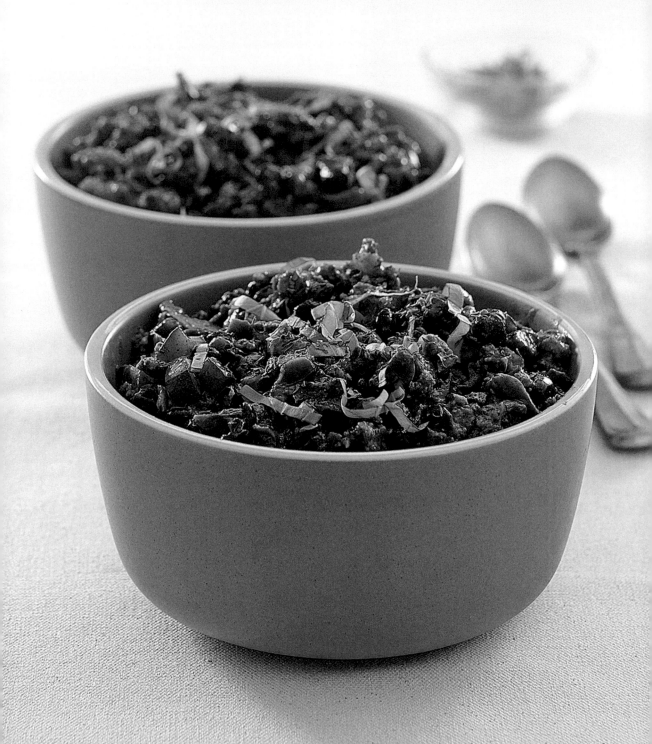

# Herb-Seasoned Hearty Turkey Chili

*This is one of my favorite winter recipes. It is full of flavor, easy to make, and plenty nutritious. You can eat it as is, over rice, with a layer of shredded cheese, or with a dollop of sour cream. You can also swap in and out different types of beans like white beans and chickpeas, which are all a great source of metabolism-supporting soluble fiber. Another option is to try it with ground beef or chicken or even take out the meat entirely for a satisfying meatless meal. Whatever you don't eat within 2–3 days can be frozen for later.*

2 tablespoons extra-virgin olive oil

½ medium red onion, chopped

5 cloves garlic, chopped

1 pound 93 percent lean ground turkey

1 (28-ounce) can diced tomatoes

2 cups baby bella (cremini) mushrooms, diced

1 small zucchini, diced

1½ cups canned kidney beans, drained and rinsed

1½ cups canned black beans, drained and rinsed

2 teaspoons chili powder

⅛ teaspoon salt

1 teaspoon ground turmeric

2 tablespoons chopped fresh basil

2 tablespoons chopped fresh parsley

1. Heat oil in a large pot over medium heat, and then add in onion. Sauté until onion is translucent, 5–6 minutes, and then add in garlic. Sauté for 1 minute, and then add in turkey. Cook until all sides are browned.
2. Add in remaining ingredients except basil and parsley. Bring to a boil, and then reduce heat to low and simmer for 20–30 minutes.
3. Serve in individual bowls, topped with basil and parsley.

**CORE 3 SERVINGS**

1 carb
2 proteins
1 fat

**SERVES**
4

**NUTRITION FACTS PER SERVING**

| | |
|---|---|
| Calories: | 465 |
| **Fiber:** | **16g** |
| Carbohydrates: | 44g |
| Sugar: | 7g |
| Protein: | 35g |
| Fat: | 16g |
| Sodium: | 881mg |

**NOTE**
Keep in mind this recipe is higher in sodium. If you have a history of high blood pressure, or need to watch sodium intake for other reasons, I recommend only enjoying on occasion.

**SERVES**

2

**NUTRITION FACTS
PER SERVING**

| | |
|---|---|
| Calories: | 332 |
| **Fiber:** | **4g** |
| Carbohydrates: | 14g |
| Sugar: | 4g |
| Protein: | 24g |
| Fat: | 22g |
| Sodium: | 853mg |

# Sesame Ginger Tofu & Veggies

*Whether you're vegan or not, incorporating more plant-powered proteins can introduce a wider range of nutrients. Tofu is a complete source of protein, with all nine essential amino acids, and a leading source of bone-protecting calcium, blood-pumping iron, energizing B vitamins, and oxidative stress–fighting selenium. It makes a worthy addition to any meal plan and can be enjoyed cooked (as in this recipe) or added uncooked to salads and smoothies for a creamy boost of protein.*

1 tablespoon extra-virgin olive oil

1 (16-ounce) package tofu, cubed

2 cups chopped baby bella (cremini) mushrooms

3 cloves garlic, minced

3 tablespoons low-sodium soy sauce

¼ teaspoon ground ginger

⅛ teaspoon salt

2 cups raw spinach

1 tablespoon sesame oil

1 tablespoon chopped fresh parsley

2 scallions, diced

1. Heat olive oil in a large skillet over medium heat. Add in tofu and cook for 4–5 minutes, stirring frequently.
2. Add in mushrooms and garlic. Cook for another 3–4 minutes, and then add in soy sauce, ginger, and salt. Cook for another 2 minutes, and then stir in spinach and sesame oil. Cook until spinach starts to wilt, 1–2 minutes, and then remove from pan and garnish with parsley and scallions.

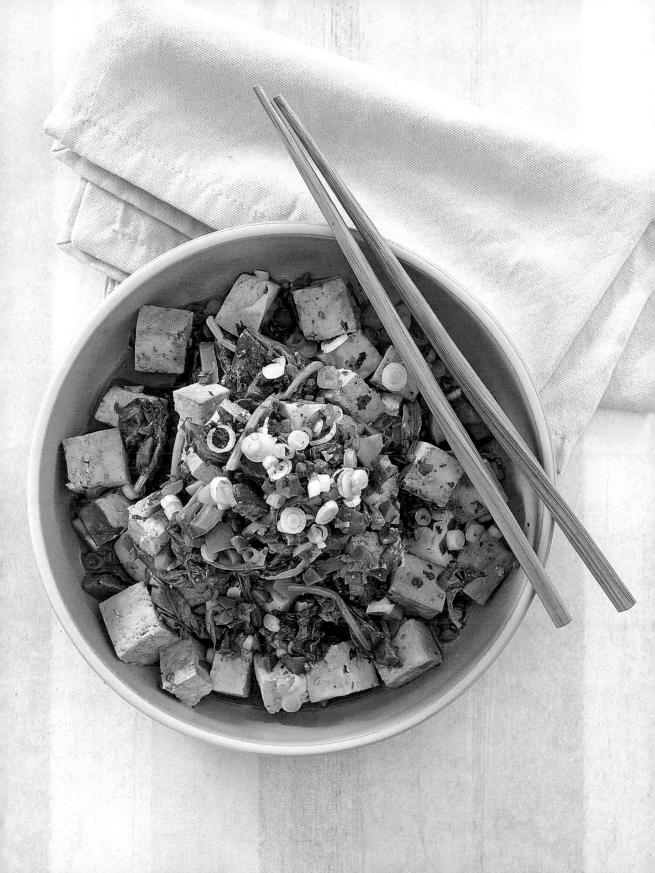

**CORE 3 SERVINGS**

2 carbs
2 proteins
1 fat

**SERVES**
1

**NUTRITION FACTS
PER SERVING**

| | |
|---|---|
| Calories: | 533 |
| **Fiber:** | **34g** |
| Carbohydrates: | 80g |
| Sugar: | 11g |
| Protein: | 33g |
| Fat: | 10g |
| Sodium: | 1,320mg |

**NOTE**

Keep in mind this recipe is higher in sodium. If you have a history of high blood pressure, or need to watch sodium intake for other reasons, I recommend using low-sodium canned beans and omitting the salsa.

# Vegan Burrito Bowl

*This 100 percent vegan burrito bowl is packed with nutrients from A to zinc. It's also a great source of fiber and can be enjoyed as an energizing lunch or a quick dinner. What I love about this dish is that it requires only a few simple ingredients and yet it tastes like you spent hours making it.*

2 teaspoons extra-virgin olive oil

¼ cup chopped white onion

1 cup riced cauliflower

¼ teaspoon garlic powder

1½ cups canned black beans, drained and rinsed

½ cup cherry tomatoes, halved

¼ cup nutritional yeast

¼ cup jarred salsa

1 tablespoon chopped fresh cilantro

1. Heat oil in a large skillet over medium heat. Add onion and stir for 5–10 minutes, until softened. Add cauliflower and stir for 1–2 minutes. Cover and cook for 5–8 minutes, until tender. Remove from heat and let cool, and then transfer to a bowl.
2. Mix in garlic powder. Top with beans, tomatoes, nutritional yeast, and salsa. Garnish with cilantro.

# Hearty Chicken Minestrone Soup

*This soup is another way to use the chicken and strained broth made in the Easy Chicken Veggie Soup recipe (see recipe in this chapter). Soups can be enjoyed as an appetizer, side, or a main course and it contains all essential Core Three nutrients. To turn this soup completely plant-based, simply omit the chicken and use vegetable broth. It can be eaten as a standalone meal or as an appetizer. You can also add grated Parmesan cheese on top.*

**CORE 3 SERVINGS**
1 carb
2 proteins
1 fat

**SERVES**
4

**NUTRITION FACTS PER SERVING**

| | |
|---|---|
| Calories: | 432 |
| **Fiber:** | **13g** |
| Carbohydrates: | 46g |
| Sugar: | 10g |
| Protein: | 36g |
| Fat: | 10g |
| Sodium: | 1,469mg |

**NOTE**
Keep in mind this recipe is higher in sodium. If you have a history of high blood pressure, or need to watch sodium intake for other reasons, I recommend only enjoying on occasion.

- 2 tablespoons extra-virgin olive oil
- 1 medium yellow onion, finely diced
- 2 large carrots, halved lengthwise and sliced
- 3 stalks celery, sliced
- 1 large zucchini, halved lengthwise and sliced
- 1 cup raw trimmed chopped green beans
- ½ teaspoon ground black pepper
- 4 cloves garlic, minced
- 1½ teaspoons Italian seasoning
- 1 (28-ounce) can diced tomatoes
- 6 cups low-sodium chicken broth
- 2 bay leaves
- 1 (15-ounce) can kidney beans, drained and rinsed
- ½ cup uncooked whole-wheat macaroni
- 2 cups shredded cooked chicken
- 2 tablespoons chopped fresh parsley
- 1 tablespoon chopped fresh basil

1. Heat oil in a large pot over medium heat. Add onion, carrots, celery, zucchini, and green beans. Season with pepper. Cook, stirring occasionally, until vegetables start to soften, 4–5 minutes.
2. Add garlic and cook for an additional 30 seconds. Add Italian seasoning, tomatoes, and broth to the pot. Stir in bay leaves. Reduce heat to low and simmer for 20 minutes.
3. Add in beans and pasta. Cook for another 4–5 minutes, and then add chicken and cook for an additional 2–3 minutes. Garnish with parsley and basil.

**SERVES**
8

**NUTRITION FACTS
PER SERVING**

| | |
|---|---|
| Calories: | 101 |
| **Fiber:** | **1g** |
| Carbohydrates: | 6g |
| Sugar: | 2g |
| Protein: | 12g |
| Fat: | 3g |
| Sodium: | 930mg |

**NOTE**

Keep in mind this recipe is higher in sodium. If you have a history of high blood pressure, or need to watch sodium intake for other reasons, I recommend only enjoying on occasion.

# Easy Chicken Veggie Soup

*Soup is a seasonal comfort food that can be an incredibly nutritious and filling option. Broth contains tons of immune-balancing nutrients like zinc, vitamin C, and phytonutrients that fight inflammation. There are so many options when it comes to soup add-ins, so feel free to toss in more than what I've listed here. If you don't eat chicken, you can omit it from the recipe.*

1 (4-pound) whole raw chicken, cut into pieces
4 medium carrots, sliced crosswise ¼ inch thick
4 stalks celery, sliced crosswise ¼ inch thick
1 medium white onion, thinly sliced
4 cloves garlic, crushed
3 bay leaves
3 tablespoons chopped fresh parsley
8 cups water
3 teaspoons salt
1 tablespoon lemon juice

1. Add all ingredients to a large pot and bring to a boil. Reduce heat to low and simmer for at least 45 minutes and up to 2 hours.
2. Before eating soup, strain it to remove all bones and roughage. You can then slice carrots and chicken and put them back into the broth, or you can discard all solid parts and use the broth as a base for other soup recipes.
3. After refrigerating, skim and discard the top, as the fat will rise to the surface and harden.

# Chicken Spinach Artichoke Spaghetti Squash

*Spaghetti squash can replace pasta in any of your favorite recipes, and you can top it with any type of sauce. Spaghetti squash is nutritious and satisfying, and it will help you easily reach your minimum of three veggie servings per day.*

**CORE 3 SERVINGS**
1 carb
1 protein
2 fats

**SERVES**
3

**NUTRITION FACTS PER SERVING**

| | |
|---|---|
| Calories: | 378 |
| **Fiber:** | **6g** |
| Carbohydrates: | 32g |
| Sugar: | 13g |
| Protein: | 27g |
| Fat: | 17g |
| Sodium: | 616mg |

1 medium spaghetti squash

2 tablespoons extra-virgin olive oil, divided

¼ teaspoon salt, divided

½ medium yellow onion, chopped

8 ounces raw boneless, skinless chicken breast, cut into cubes

4 cloves garlic, chopped

¼ teaspoon red pepper flakes

1 (14-ounce) can artichoke hearts, drained

2 cups raw spinach

¾ cup cherry tomatoes, sliced

½ cup whole-milk Greek yogurt

¼ cup grated Parmesan cheese

⅓ cup grated part-skim mozzarella cheese

1. Preheat oven to 400°F.
2. Microwave squash for 5 minutes. Slice in half and scrape out just the seeds to discard. Drizzle with 2 teaspoons oil and season with ⅛ teaspoon salt. Transfer to a parchment paper–lined baking sheet, with outside or skinned side facing up, and poke a few holes in squash with a fork. Bake for 30 minutes.
3. While squash is cooking, heat remaining 4 teaspoons oil in a large skillet over medium heat. Add onion, cook for about 5 minutes, and then add in chicken and garlic. Cook until lightly browned, and then add in red pepper flakes, artichoke hearts, spinach, tomatoes, yogurt, Parmesan, and remaining salt. Stir until spinach is softened, 2–3 minutes.
4. Remove squash from oven and scrape with a fork until strands are loosened, resembling spaghetti. Leave strands in squash shell. Divide chicken and veggies between squash halves, top with mozzarella, and bake for another 5–10 minutes, until mozzarella is melted.
5. Scoop out into bowls and enjoy.

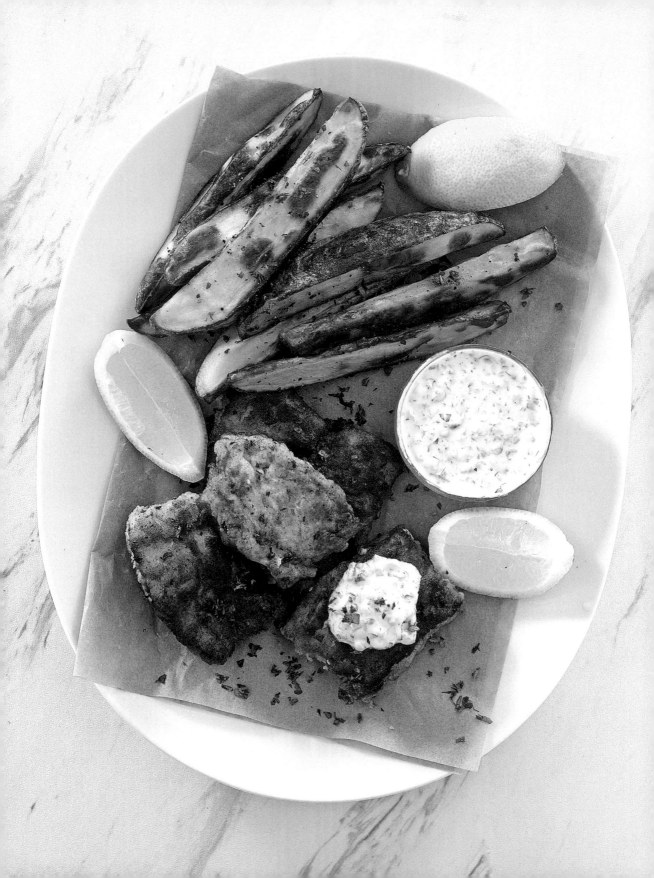

# Air-Fried Fish & Chips

*If you don't own an air fryer, you can bake the fish and chips in the oven at 400°F for 10–12 minutes. You can replace the cod with haddock, sole, sea bass, or halibut.*

**CORE 3 SERVINGS**

1 carb
1 protein
2 fats

### Fish and Chips

4 small russet potatoes

2 tablespoons extra-virgin olive oil, divided

1/8 teaspoon sea salt, divided

1/4 teaspoon ground black pepper, divided

4 (4-ounce) cod fillets

2 large eggs

2/3 cup almond flour

2 tablespoons psyllium husk powder

1/2 teaspoon garlic powder

1/4 teaspoon paprika

1/4 teaspoon dried parsley

Olive oil spray

### Greek Yogurt Tartar Sauce

1/2 cup plain full-fat Greek yogurt

1 teaspoon Dijon mustard

2 tablespoons finely diced dill pickles

1 tablespoon finely diced capers

1/8 teaspoon dried dill

**SERVES**
4

**NUTRITION FACTS PER SERVING (1 FISH FILLET, 1 POTATO, AND 1/4 OF DIPPING SAUCE)**

| | |
|---|---|
| Calories: | 440 |
| **Fiber:** | **9g** |
| Carbohydrates: | 38g |
| Sugar: | 3g |
| Protein: | 30g |
| Fat: | 18g |
| Sodium: | 973mg |

**NOTE**
Keep in mind this recipe is higher in sodium. If you have a history of high blood pressure, or need to watch sodium intake for other reasons, I recommend only enjoying on occasion.

1. For the Fish and Chips: Preheat oven to 400°F.
2. Cut potatoes into wedges. In a large bowl, toss potatoes with 1 tablespoon oil and half of salt and pepper. Transfer to a baking sheet and bake for 25–30 minutes.
3. While potatoes are cooking, pat fish dry. Crack eggs into a shallow bowl and mix until frothy. In a medium bowl, mix flour, psyllium husk, garlic powder, paprika, parsley, and remaining salt and pepper. Working with one fillet at a time, coat fish in eggs, and then dip each side in flour mixture until coated.
4. Add remaining 1 tablespoon oil to air fryer, and then place fish inside. Cook at 390°F for 14–15 minutes. After the first 8 minutes, flip the fillets and spray with oil. Continue cooking for the remaining time.
5. For the Greek Yogurt Tartar Sauce: While fish is cooking, mix all ingredients in a small bowl.
6. Remove fish from air fryer and serve with potatoes and a side of tartar sauce.

## Shrimp "Fried Rice"

**SERVES**
4

**NUTRITION FACTS
PER SERVING**

| | |
|---|---|
| Calories: | 286 |
| **Fiber:** | **4g** |
| Carbohydrates: | 13g |
| Sugar: | 3g |
| Protein: | 24g |
| Fat: | 15g |
| Sodium: | 906mg |

**NOTE**
Keep in mind this recipe is higher in sodium. If you have a history of high blood pressure, or need to watch sodium intake for other reasons, I recommend only enjoying on occasion.

*Contrary to popular belief, shrimp is not a cholesterol-spiking food. It does have dietary cholesterol, but as discussed in Chapter 6, dietary saturated fat is the biggest culprit behind elevated LDL cholesterol, and omega-6s can more be detrimental to heart health. Shrimp is also a good source of selenium (which is needed for thyroid hormone production), anti-inflammatory omega-3s, energy-boosting B12, and choline (which is important for mood, memory, and muscle control).*

2 tablespoons coconut oil, divided

1 pound raw shrimp, peeled, deveined, and chopped

1 tablespoon chopped fresh ginger

4 cloves garlic, sliced

4 medium scallions, thinly sliced, whites and greens separated

4 cups frozen riced cauliflower

1 cup frozen peas and carrots

2 large eggs, beaten

2 tablespoons chopped peanuts

¼ teaspoon crushed red pepper flakes

1 tablespoons tamari

1 tablespoon unseasoned rice vinegar

1 tablespoon sesame oil

1. Heat 1 tablespoon coconut oil in a large skillet over medium-high heat. Add shrimp and cook for 4–6 minutes. Remove from pan and set aside.
2. Add remaining 1 tablespoon coconut oil, ginger, garlic, and scallion whites to pan. Cook, stirring, until fragrant, about 1 minute.
3. Pour in cauliflower, peas, and carrots and stir for 4–5 minutes.
4. Crack eggs on top of cauliflower mixture and quickly stir for about 1 minute.
5. Return shrimp to pan and mix well. Add scallion greens, peanuts, red pepper flakes, tamari, vinegar, and sesame oil. Serve.

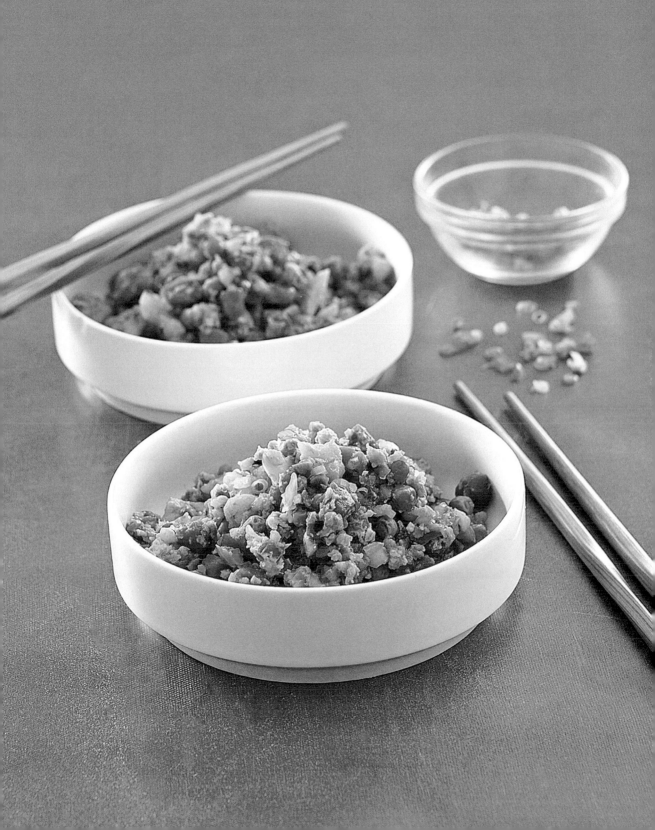

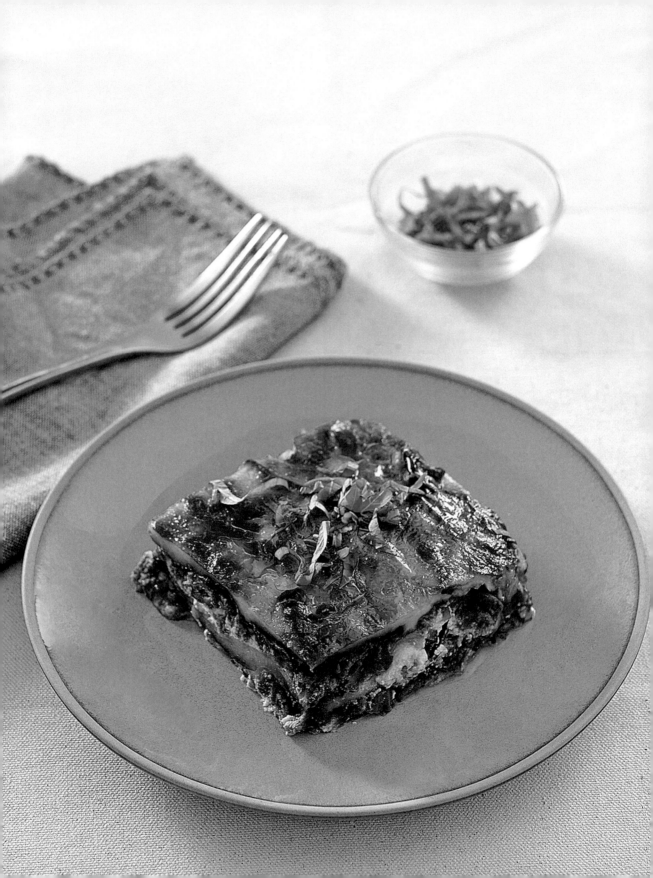

# Very Veggie Lasagna

*Replacing pasta with thinly sliced eggplant and zucchini is an easy approach for getting in more veggies and fiber and naturally decreasing carb intake. You can also still incorporate traditional lasagna noodles, but alternate layers using one strip of pasta, one strip of eggplant or zucchini, and so on. If you prefer beef, try to use grass-fed ground beef. This can last a few days or be stored in the freezer for a later time. If you don't eat meat or follow a kosher diet, you can simply omit the turkey.*

1 medium purple eggplant, sliced thin lengthwise

1½ tablespoons salt, divided

4 tablespoons extra-virgin olive oil, divided

½ medium white onion, chopped

1 pound 93 percent lean ground turkey

4 cloves garlic, chopped

1 (24-ounce) jar tomato sauce

1 medium zucchini, sliced thin lengthwise

12 ounces part-skim ricotta cheese

1 large egg

1 cup shredded part-skim mozzarella cheese

3 tablespoons chopped fresh basil, divided

2 tablespoons chopped fresh parsley, divided

*continued*

**CORE 3 SERVINGS**

0 carb
1 protein
2½ fats

**SERVES**
6

**NUTRITION FACTS PER SERVING**

| | |
|---|---|
| Calories: | 428 |
| **Fiber:** | **4g** |
| Carbohydrates: | 18g |
| Sugar: | 9g |
| Protein: | 28g |
| Fat: | 26g |
| Sodium: | 1,117mg |

**NOTE**

Keep in mind this recipe is higher in sodium. If you have a history of high blood pressure, or need to watch sodium intake for other reasons, I recommend only enjoying on occasion.

1. Preheat oven to 400°F.
2. Soak eggplant in 8 cups water with 1 tablespoon salt for 20–30 minutes—this helps remove some of the bitterness and excess liquid. Place a pot or an upside-down plate on top to keep eggplant fully submerged.
3. Heat 2 tablespoons oil in a large pot over medium heat. Add in onion and stir until translucent, 5–7 minutes. Add in turkey, garlic, and remaining ½ tablespoon salt. Stir until meat is browned on all sides, 7–10 minutes. Pour tomato sauce on top and bring to a boil. Reduce heat to low and simmer for 15–20 minutes.
4. Heat 1 tablespoon oil in a large skillet over medium heat. Lay eggplant in pan and cook on each side for 2–3 minutes or until softened. Repeat with zucchini and remaining 1 tablespoon oil.
5. In a medium bowl, mix ricotta with egg.
6. In an oven-safe casserole dish, arrange half of zucchini on the bottom, then layer on half of ricotta and egg mixture, half of meat sauce, half of eggplant, half of mozzarella, 1 tablespoon basil, and 1 tablespoon parsley. Layer remaining zucchini on top of mozzarella and repeat with remaining ricotta, meat sauce, eggplant, and mozzarella. Finish with 1 tablespoon basil and remaining 1 tablespoon parsley.
7. Cook for 40–45 minutes, and then broil for 5 minutes for a crispier top. Garnish with remaining 1 tablespoon basil.

# Zesty Grilled Fish Tacos

*This recipe packs in plenty of antioxidants from the cabbage, olive oil, and seasonings. You can enjoy the fish, sauce, and slaw in a soft- or hard-shell taco or over a bed of mixed greens. If you can't find cod, halibut, mahi-mahi, or snapper would also work well.*

## Tacos

1 pound cod

1/8 teaspoon salt

1/8 teaspoon ground black pepper

1 tablespoon extra-virgin olive oil

Juice from 1 small lime

2 cloves garlic, chopped

1 teaspoon ground cumin

1 teaspoon paprika

1/4 teaspoon cayenne pepper

8 (6-inch) whole-wheat tortillas

1 medium avocado, diced

## Taco Sauce

1/2 cup full-fat Greek yogurt

Juice from 1 small lime

1/2 teaspoon garlic powder

1 teaspoon sriracha

1 1/2 teaspoons avocado oil

## Cabbage Slaw

4 cups shredded purple cabbage

1 tablespoon Dijon mustard

1 teaspoon extra-virgin olive oil

1 tablespoon honey

1 tablespoon apple cider vinegar

1/8 teaspoon salt

1/4 teaspoon ground black pepper

1 1/2 teaspoons lemon juice

**CORE 3 SERVINGS**

1 carb

2 proteins

1 1/2 fats

**SERVES**

4

**NUTRITION FACTS PER SERVING**

| | |
|---|---|
| Calories: | 492 |
| **Fiber:** | **10g** |
| Carbohydrates: | 58g |
| Sugar: | 14g |
| Protein: | 28g |
| Fat: | 17g |
| Sodium: | 962mg |

**NOTE**

Keep in mind this recipe is higher in sodium. If you have a history of high blood pressure, or need to watch sodium intake for other reasons, I recommend only enjoying on occasion.

*continued*

1. For the Tacos: Pat fish dry and sprinkle salt and pepper on each side.
2. In a small bowl, combine oil, lime juice, garlic, cumin, paprika, and cayenne.
3. Place fish and marinade in a large zip-top bag and let marinate in fridge for 20–30 minutes.
4. For the Taco Sauce: While fish is marinating, combine all sauce ingredients in a small bowl.
5. For the Cabbage Slaw: In a large bowl, combine all slaw ingredients.
6. Heat grill to medium heat and brush with oil. Grill each side of fish for 3–4 minutes, depending on the type and thickness of fish. Transfer to plate before breaking up into smaller pieces.
7. Add tortillas to grill and warm for a few seconds.
8. Lay out tortillas on a plate and top with fish, sauce, and avocado. Sprinkle slaw on top or serve on the side.

# Index